Praise for Erica Tucci and Her Books

For RADIANT SURVIVOR

"Erica Tucci touches on a subject I am all too well aware of. Her story is mine. She brings the reader through the realities and frustrations of suffering a life-threatening illness but adds that ray of light at the end of that dark tunnel, as hope is always there if you believe and find your own true strength."
~ **KEVIN SORBO**
Actor, Director, Producer, and Author of *True Strength*

"Survivors have common qualities and are an excellent resource for all of us. They become our life coaches and help us to learn from our experiences and be guided by them. Erica's experience can help us all to learn about survivor behavior and thriving in difficult times."
~ **BERNIE SIEGEL, MD**
Author of *A Book of Miracles* and *The Art of Healing*

"All of us face challenges, but it's the grace and wisdom we bring to those challenges that define us. Erica's search for the deeper meaning and spiritual wisdom behind her life-altering stroke sets her apart as a 'wisdom teacher' for the rest of us. This book offers a contemplative guide for anyone going through a life crisis."
~ **SUE FREDERICK**
Author of *Bridges to Heaven: True Stories of Loved Ones on the Other Side* and *I See Your Dream Job*

"Recovery from a traumatic situation in one's life can be a formidable challenge. Erica Tucci's book Radiant Survivor provides the reader with the physical, emotional and spiritual support needed to help anyone facing tragedy or overwhelming personal challenge in their

lives. It offers a beam of sunshine that, although recovery may be difficult, one can survive and thrive amidst the chaos."

~ **MAL DUANE**

Author of *Alpha Chick: Five Step for Moving from Pain to Power*

"*Radiant Survivor* is well-written and very informative. It would certainly benefit anyone whose life has been touched by stress or illness. Erica clearly gives us techniques and tips on how to reduce our stress and live a healthier lifestyle. I would highly recommend reading this book, as your life can only improve."

~ **KAREN WHITELAW-SMITH**

Speaker, Coach and Author of *The Butterfly Experience: How to Transform Your Life from the Inside Out*

"*Radiant Survivor* does a wonderful job presenting a holistic perspective on healing and moving forward. Ms. Tucci conveys a common theme of perseverance and being open to possibilities throughout the book that inspires and reminds us to believe in the power of transformation and healing both physically and emotionally. As a bonus, the exercises at the end of chapters are great ideas to jumpstart our transformation. This is a fantastic book to inspire anyone in your life!"

~ **DR. ERICA KOSAL**

Resilience expert and author of *Miracles for Daddy: A Family's Inspirational Fight against a Modern Medical Goliath*

For ANYTHING IS POSSIBLE

"*Anything is Possible* is an engaging narrative of a life and love lived in accordance with one's own feminine inner journey. It is the story not only of an adventure embracing one's difficulty of external life, but of confronting the inner complexities of one's inner life, as well. It is the story that every woman should come to realize."

~ **DR NANCY QUALLS-CORBETT**

Jungian Analyst and Author of *The Sacred Prostitute*

"I found reading the book to be a delicious experience like drinking hot chocolate in front of a cozy winter fire."
~ SAQI DOSAJ
www.wonderfulreadings.com

"Erica's story was so down-to-earth and easy to relate to. Her writing flows so effortlessly, I felt like I was living through it with her. But she kept me wondering what was going to happen next. She made me realize that if you really want something in life, you can make it happen."
~ D. L. BRIGGS

"What a beautiful read! All these years I have been in love with the author Joy Fielding. Now I have you to admire. You have the creative gift. I hope there are other projects in the works. A talent such as yours should not be left stagnant. Keep the creative juices flowing! I hope I will be the first to get your next edition when it comes out."
~ T. FERRARA

"What a luscious mystical tale Erica has written about two people living oceans apart and yet connected deeply in spirit. Theirs is a love so profound and with such passion, yet it must stand the test of time and transformation. As the novel is so appropriately entitled, Anything Is Possible!"
~ ANTOINETTE AND RICHARD ASIMUS
Founders of www.TantraHeart.com

For ZESTY WOMANHOOD AT 40 and BEYOND

"Such a glorious way of expressing the renewal of feminine power that our world is experiencing. Zesty Womanhood at 40 and Beyond is a delightfully exciting collection of observations about the 40-something woman who joyfully ventures into the next season of her life to find the treasures that await her."
~ ANTOINETTE AND RICHARD ASIMUS
Founders of www.TantraHeart.com

"There is a rising balance between the Yin and the Yang in the world through the increasing emergence of feminine energy and wisdom. Erica Tucci has captured this evolution beautifully in her book Zesty Womanhood at 40 and Beyond as she reveals how her own personal experiences as a woman returning to her center of power are a reflection of many women at the same crossroads in life."

~ **RACHAEL JAYNE GROOVER**

Founder of The Yin Project

Author of *Powerful and Feminine: How to Increase Your Magnetic Presence and Attract the Attention You Want*

ERICA TUCCI

Radiant Survivor

HOW TO SHINE & THRIVE THROUGH RECOVERY
FROM STROKE, CANCER, ABUSE, ADDICTION
AND OTHER LIFE-ALTERING EXPERIENCES

The Total Transformation of Self

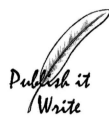

Publish It Write
14315 Lost Meadow
Houston, Texas 77079
832.335.0272

www.ericatucci.com

Text copyright © 2013 by Erica Tucci

Cover design by Renee Duran
Interior design by Lynn Serafinn
Text editing and proofing by Vrinda Pendred

Edition ISBNs
Softcover – 978-0-9662451-7-2
e-book – 978-0-9662451-6-5

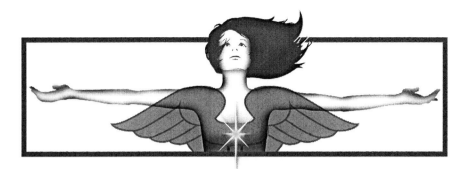

Table of Contents

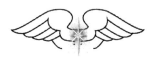

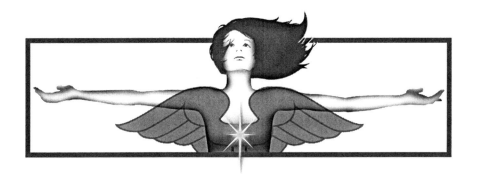

Acknowledgments

Writing this book was an act of love for those of you who I hope will be touched by its messages and lifted up from fear and despair to hope and radiance. And as I was writing it, I discovered that as I was hopefully helping you with my words, I was also healing myself. As we become agents of change for others, so too are we transformed.

I want to acknowledge all those who helped make this book metamorphose from just an idea in my head of simply telling my story to a collection of compelling stories and pearls of wisdom. These have come from others who faced similar life-altering experiences to my own, as well as from caregivers who faced their own set of challenges in taking care of their charges. Thank you all story contributors for making this book shine so brightly.

Much gratitude goes to the fabulous marketing team led by Lynn Serafinn, for the phenomenal job they did bringing this book to market. This includes Renee Duran, the graphic designer who created a book cover that perfectly conveyed the underlying message of the book.

And I certainly can't forget my editor, Vrinda Pendred, who did a magnificent job of tightening my wordiness so that my messages were clear.

But none of this brilliance could have happened without the wonderful support of my friends and family, especially my mom who cared for me throughout my rehabilitation, providing a safe haven in which I could fully recover.

Nor could I have done it without the support of the donors who so graciously contributed to my funding campaign so I could actually publish my book: Howard Batt, Sarah Bronson, Kim Crabb, Phil Morabito, Janie Nguyen, Dr. Bart Putterman, Aurelio Sablone, Saqi Salehi, Robin Swanger, Mark Wilkinson and many others.

My deepest appreciation to all of you for making this book real and, thus, transforming my life. I am a better person because of it.

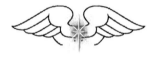

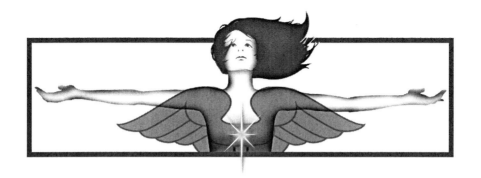

Introduction

H ave you ever faced a situation that completely changed your life, one that may have brought you to the brink of death, be it physical or emotional, only to transform you from the person you were to a person with a whole new set of beliefs, values and truths? Mine happened June 10, 2011 at 6:30 am.

But before I tell you my story, I want to tell you why I'm so glad you've chosen to read my book. As you might have already gathered from the title, it's a book of transformation, moving from the old to the new. I hope you see it as a resource for your own healing, as well as a vehicle through which you can help others, if you choose to do so.

At the time I began writing this introduction, I was 85% recovered from my trauma, after months and months of rehab, exercise, massage, Reiki, yoga and any other modalities I could use to heal my body. As much as I have done, it seems I will actually be better than before. I am on the road to full recovery and I hope that before I finish writing this book, I will have completed my metamorphosis into the person I am meant to be, instead of the person I was, not only physically but, most importantly, emotionally and spiritually. I will have healed, at least from the life circumstance that was brought into the light during this odyssey.

Our healing never stops, not as long as we live in our physical bodies. What I desire now is to use my healing experience and share it with others, in hopes that my transformation into the person I will be will help others see their own life-changing circumstances not as a curse but a blessing. Life challenges are truly gifts from the soul, offering so many opportunities to grow as we learn the lessons we are being taught, and to gain wisdom from these lessons. And because there are so many different types of trauma we can face in this world, my story being only one, I have also included others' stories of their tragedies and victories – breast cancer, loss of a loved one, emotional and sexual abuse, addiction, depression leading to feelings of suicide, and others...very compelling and powerful indeed! You will also find stories from caregivers, as they too are affected in many ways. (Note that the stories are written using either American or British English, depending on the story contributor's place of residence.)

Please note that each chapter is written with different underlying emotions and perspectives. As I went through the different phases of my recovery, the theme of each chapter was what I needed to work on at the moment of writing it. These are reflected in my own experiences, as well as in the diverse testimonials used to elucidate the various themes. They all had a unique effect on me: some are heavy with story, some are more weighted with pearls of wisdom and others have a balance between both.

Beyond my story, the subsequent chapters of this book explore the various perspectives of recovery from life-altering experiences, addressing such subjects as:

- Believing in yourself and never giving up
- Understanding the limiting beliefs that hold you back from being all you can be
- Being grateful and having the right attitude

- Knowing that your experience is part of your sacred contract with the Divine
- Surrendering and letting go
- Establishing your support system
- Seeing recovery as a process
- Wondering what to do if you don't fully recover
- Finding out what's really important in life
- The caregiver's perspective

...and more!

This book is both spiritual and practical; as we are spiritual beings living in physical bodies, we must live life from the soul, but with a certain amount of logical reasoning. There may be parts that challenge your beliefs or discuss topics you've never thought about. All I ask is that you open your mind to all possibilities, as it is with this "receptivity" that new and wonderful opportunities in life can flourish and bring you to a greater level of awareness of life itself.

I do hope what you read in the pages of this book is most useful to you in living through any difficult circumstances. I've tried to sprinkle the stories and discussions with bits of humor. I've also included exercises at the end of each chapter to reflect on your situation and help you ensure that everything possible is done for your healing. So have a journal or notebook handy.

Life is not meant to be hard. It's meant to be full of joy and peace, even in the roughest of times. "You can use a challenge to awaken you, or you can allow it to pull you into even darker sleep."[1] I truly believe our attitudes either awaken us to all possibilities in life or they can plunge us into a dark abyss. Where would you rather be?

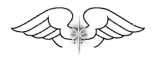

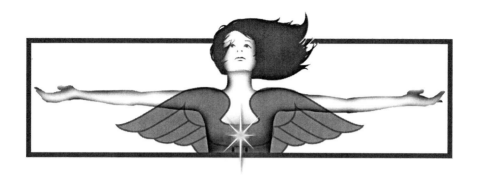

My Story

That very memorable morning, I woke up as always at 5:00 to meditate, perform my morning exercises, shower and eat breakfast before getting ready for work. As I stepped out of my bedroom and into my living room, purse flung over my shoulder and car keys in hand, ready to head out the door, something strange happened. I collapsed onto the floor. No warning, no signs, no symptoms...just a simple belly flop onto the carpeted floor. Figure that one out! I sure couldn't! And no matter how hard I tried to get up, my body just wouldn't cooperate. It seemed like my body was no longer whole, like a part was missing.

I don't know how long I struggled to get up with the operable part of my body before giving up and turning over on my back, but when I did, I realized something was terribly wrong. I lay there for a moment, contemplating the situation. I was completely coherent, my mind filled with mixed thoughts of wonder and disbelief. What had just happened? Why was I lying in the middle of my living room floor, unable to get up? What did I do?

My 19-year old son (at the time) was in his bedroom just 10 feet away, but I couldn't yell. My vocal cords seemed frozen. When I fell, my purse had fallen with me – lucky for me. With my hand that was still working, I took my phone out of my purse and dialed my mom's number. Three rings and...

"Hello," sounded at the other end.

"Mumm." It took every bit of effort to get that one word out.

"Erica...is that you?" Mom asked, recognizing the phone number on her cell phone. "What's wrong?" I could sense panic in her voice.

"I dun no wat's 'appenin'." I could barely talk; my mouth felt numb, my words slurring.

Mom's worry intensified over the phone. "My God, where's Brett?"

"Call 'im. He's in 'is room."

My son didn't keep his phone on while he slept, and he usually slept until noon (since it was summer and he was out of school). But as fate would have it, he had his phone on that morning. I heard his phone ring and, within minutes, he came running out of his room.

"Mom, what happened?" my son questioned as he called 911, his eyes as big as saucers. "Please send an ambulance!" he blurted into the phone. "I think my mom's had a stroke!"

It was kind of a blur from then until the ambulance arrived, only minutes later. I was actually surprised at how quickly they came, but I soon found out why. If a stroke victim is administered a tPA (tissue plasminogen activator) within three hours of having a stroke, the effects of the stroke can be minimized substantially. In my case, I had an ischemic stroke (caused by a blood clot) that affected my basal ganglia, which controls voluntary motor control and cognitive and emotional functions. Since I arrived at the hospital in time, they were able to administer the tPA, thus reducing the consequences of my condition. Of course, there was also the risk of me dying from the medication and I had to sign a release before they would administer it. But I was willing to take the risk and signed. Lucky for me, I didn't die!

Regarding the effects of the stroke, I still had my wits about me, although I did tend to forget things (of course, I was forgetful even before my illness!), and I was pretty emotional (but again, I've always been very emotional and I am of menopausal age, so who knows if the stroke exacerbated my emotions?). Mom and I laughed at my behavior after the stroke because anything could trigger tears, although it was usually very short-lived; it was only seconds before I bounced back. Most affected were my motor skills. I became a hemiplegic, where the right side of my body was completely paralyzed. In the hospital, I couldn't even lift a finger.

Well, while I was trekking to the hospital in the ambulance, Mom was "flying" in her car as fast as she could, as if she was on a broomstick, running stop signs she didn't even see, with her focus on getting to the hospital as soon as possible. I guess the cops were on vacation at the time, or maybe Spirit cloaked Mom's car in an invisible wrap so they couldn't see her. She got to my apartment, where Brett was waiting for her, and the two of them raced to the hospital.

After going to the emergency room, then to the ICU where they ran what seemed like hundreds of tests, I finally landed in my own hospital room with numerous wires running from me to all the machines they had me hooked up to. I looked like the Bride of Frankenstein. And that is where the fun began, starting with the most fundamental question....

Why Did It Happen?

I was seemingly in great condition. I was slender, I worked out at least three times a week, and I had none of the risk factors such as high blood pressure or high cholesterol. There weren't any hereditary heart conditions in my family. So why did I have a stroke? Yes, I was working 80+ hours a week, since I was a corporate manager at a Fortune 500 company while trying to build a healing arts business on the side, as well as writing and publishing two books. My foray into massage, Reiki, life coaching and writing was my true passion and, one day, I hoped to do only that, leaving my life as a corporate cog behind me in the dust. Yes, I was stressed out working so many hours, but I loved what I was doing and couldn't name my stress as the culprit. There had to be something more to it.

During the course of my recovery, little by little, the vision of the truth behind my "dis-ease" became clear. It was as much a spiritual journey as it was a physical one. The mantra I lived by was, "I am on a magic carpet ride, with Spirit at the helm." I knew there would be speed bumps, but I never knew how big they could be.

First things first: while in the ICU, one of the tests they ran on me was a trans-esophageal echocardiogram (TEE) to assess the health of my heart. Lo and behold, they found that I had a PFO (patent foramen ovale), which in simple terms means I had a hole in my heart. Actually, we're all born with one, but it's supposed to close soon after birth. Yet did you know that for 25% of humans, this hole remains open even in adulthood? There are no symptoms, and the condition is not usually treated unless there are other heart problems, or a person has a stroke caused by a blood clot.

Isn't that great? Someone has to wait until they have a life-threatening condition before they find out what caused it, something that could have been prevented by a simple test...well, I wouldn't say "simple". A TEE is by no means simple. A probe with a transducer is inserted down the esophagus, emitting ultrasonic sound waves that are sent to a computer to interpret the echoes into an image of the heart walls and valves.

Now we knew physically why I had a stroke. The hole in my heart allowed a blood clot to pass through it and settle in my brain. But the doctors were still somewhat baffled because when they checked my body for blood clots, particularly my legs, they couldn't find any others. Apparently, older people with PFOs (geez, I'm not that old!) often develop blood clots in their leg veins. The only one I had was the one that reached my brain, where it wreaked havoc on my body. I guess it only takes one!

But the bewilderment surrounding my stroke led me to seek more profound answers as to "why" this happened to me. I'm not talking about the "why me" of someone feeling like a victim of circumstance. I'm talking about the bigger "why", the underlying truth. And in my quest for the Truth, I went on the most reflective spiritual journey I'd ever been on.

Since I can remember, I have always been very introspective – meditating regularly; going on meditation retreats; reading every spiritually-oriented book that resonated with me and gleaning everything I could from them; undergoing different forms of therapy, including energy work and past-life regression – all helping me approach what I consider my Truth.

The Truth – My Truth

I was reading Dr. Brian Weiss' book *Miracles Happen: The Transformational Healing Power of Past-Life Therapies* and it reminded me of my own past-life regression sessions, which would reveal the most amazing information about my stroke. Dr. Weiss is a pioneer of past-life regression. He is a very successful psychiatrist, a graduate of Columbia University and Yale Medical School, and was Chairman Emeritus of Psychiatry at the Mount Sinai Medical Center in Miami, Florida. He was very skeptical of non-scientific fields such as reincarnation until his encounter with one of his patients, Catherine, who he regressed under hypnosis to events in her childhood that were causing the anxieties she was fraught with.

But when she went under, she took Dr. Weiss back to past lives in which she recalled memories with such vivid detail that Dr. Weiss was able to confirm some of their validity through research. She even revealed truths about Dr. Weiss that she couldn't have known without being a conduit for information from highly evolved "spirit" entities that revealed many secrets of life and death. Her past-life memories and channeled messages from the spiritual realm healed her of her anxieties within a matter of months. With these insights, Dr. Weiss' skepticism began to erode and his first book *Many Lives, Many Masters* was published in 1998, discussing his account with Catherine. He has since focused his work on past-life regression because of the tremendous healing power it has had on his patients, and he has regressed thousands since that first surprising encounter.

My first regression session actually occurred in 2009, two years before I had the debilitating episode that left my right side paralyzed. The regression took me back to 1897 in Charleston, a port in South Carolina. Before the regression, I had heard of Charleston and knew it was somewhere in the Carolinas, but I didn't know which Carolina, nor did I know it was a port.

As the regression therapist guided me back in time, she asked me, "Do you know what year it is?"

"Yes," I responded as my mind relaxed into a meditative state where our ego is set aside to allow for the flow of subconscious thoughts and images. I was lying very comfortably on her couch in her living room (she split her schedule between clients at home and clients at the center where she worked part-time). "It's 1897."

"And where are you?" she continued her enquiry.

"It looks like a port. In the Carolinas. Charleston, maybe?"

"And what are you doing?"

This is where my story took on a life of its own, revealing the past traumas that would affect me in my current life. For those of you who are skeptical about past-life regression, bear with me as I tell the story. You may find it fascinating. Plus, remember that Dr. Weiss was also a skeptic until his encounter with Catherine's story, which was far more surreal than mine.

As the therapist guided me through my life, I started out as a 12-year-old girl whose parents had died, leaving her to fend for herself. She worked at a saloon cleaning tables and sometimes serving drinks to the customers. There was a young boy around the same age, who would walk by the saloon regularly and peek in, but never enter. I knew intuitively as the observer that the youngsters had eyes for one another, but they never talked because the young boy was from a higher class than the girl and apparently his parents wouldn't let him have anything to do with her.

As the therapist brought me further into my life, the next scene was at a theatre where the girl, now in her 20s, was a well-known showgirl. A well-to-do gentleman entered as she was performing. He wore a tailored suit and spats donned his shoes, and he had an equally well-dressed woman on his left arm. As I watched the scene unfold, I saw the most unusual image. As the girl (now a young woman) danced, her eyes fell upon the well-clad couple watching her. At that moment, I saw a huge gaping hole where her heart was, as if it had been cut out, symbolically speaking. You see, the gentleman who had come in to see her perform was the same young boy from her past, the one she had kept in her heart since the first time she saw him pass by the saloon where she used to work. Needless to say, she was heartbroken at seeing him with another woman, thus the "symbolic image" of the hole in her heart.

The hole in her heart...hmmm, doesn't that sound familiar? How was I to reconcile these incidents, one in a past life and one in my current life? It wasn't until I had my stroke that I made the association between the two and decided to delve more deeply into the past life's meaning in relation to my stroke. Maybe I would have an epiphany, some nugget of wisdom that would help me find the truth behind my stroke – the cosmic truth, as we already knew the physical truth.

I had a real physical hole in my heart, but what other tidbits could I glean from that past life that would give some indication as to the karmic reason for me having a stroke? Life is based on karma. What happens in our past will most certainly affect our present life.

What Was My Karma?

In early 2012, after having my stroke, I went to another regression therapist. My first therapist, I learned, had fallen ill and was no longer working. I found another therapist who had actually trained with Dr. Weiss, which excited me to no end. I wanted to return to the same past life, to go further, to see if anything else revealed itself that would help me understand my current life predicament.

First, let me backtrack just a bit. In that first regression, the therapist tried to carry me into the later years of my life, past that night at the theatre. But it was as if there was a block in my inner vision that would let me go no further than that "heart-wrenching" scene. What I saw in my mind's eye was a painter's canvas where the upper-left corner to the lower-right corner was painted with the image of that event, particularly the hole in the heart. The remainder of the canvas was devoid of any visual expression of anything. It was as if Spirit, the Higher Powers that be, refused to let me see how the rest of the life of the girl played out. Why was I not being allowed to see the rest of her life?

I didn't find out until the next regression in 2012, when the therapist took me back to the same past life, as per my request. As I lay on the therapist's massage table in her office, covered by a blanket to keep me from getting chills and thus disrupting the session, she began by getting me to relax, just as before, in the meditative state where my ego was set aside, allowing thoughts and images to come forth. Once I was there, indicated by my fluttering eyes, she began the process of bringing me back to 1897 in Charleston so I could re-experience the life that had affected me so traumatically 114 years later. Returning to that momentous night of my performance, I wasn't prepared for what was to come!

As the therapist asked me to move forward in my life, I found myself in my backstage room undressing after the performance. I could feel a coldness in myself, a lack of emotion, as I pulled a gun from my purse. It went off and I collapsed on the floor. I had shot myself in the heart. I had been so overwrought seeing the man who had captured my heart as a young girl with another woman that I didn't want to go on living. Too much loss in my life...first both my parents, then the man who had made my heart sing.

There's another significant part to the story. First, I must reveal another facet of my current life that ties in with this past life. In 2007, I met a Belgian man through work. We fell madly in love, but there were some serious obstacles that prevented any permanence in the relationship. We spent five glorious days together when he came to visit me and, afterward, we communicated on the phone for many months. My intuition told me I had been with him before in another life, as our connection was so strong. When I shared this with him, he said, "It feels so natural. Maybe you're right about us being together before." Perhaps it was in another lifetime, or even several lifetimes, where we actually had a loving relationship. It is possible to have many lives together, as Dr. Weiss discusses in *Miracles Happen*. "Soul mates come together again and again to interact. There is karma or destiny together."[2]

However, communication slowly dwindled and finally came to a halt when we realized nothing could come of the relationship, considering the circumstances. It was a sad time in my life when I saw that my "soul mate" had left. What was really uncanny was that I had started writing a novel in 1998 (a love story) about the female protagonist's encounter with a man who was so like my Belgian. I had put the novel away after writing the synopsis and first three chapters, but picked it up again after our "chance" meeting in 2007, nine years later. I had even given the chapters to my Belgian lover for him to read, and he identified perfectly with the male protagonist. He even called me by the female protagonist's name. Had I manifested my dream of the man in 1998 into a real person in 2007? I realized the synchronicity of the situation and decided to complete the novel entitled *Anything Is Possible* in 2010.[3]

To come full circle with the story of my stroke, the Belgian man was indeed a reincarnation of the gentleman in my past life. We HAD been together before. What did it all mean? In my past life, I had committed suicide because of lost love. In my current life, I almost died from a condition that was a reflection of that profoundly emotional time. Perhaps I was being given another chance in this lifetime to reconcile the circumstances.

As if this whole discussion about past-life experiences and how it affected the present wasn't enough, there was more to my revelation of Truth as it related to my stroke. I wrote an article that I sent to my "sacred feminine community" as well as posted on my blog, entitled "Man Fears Woman – Yin Versus Yang," which gives a compelling twist to my story. I have included the article below.

"As I recover from my stroke, I have been pondering: 'Why did this happen?' Today's message is an expression of the answer to my question, not from the victim's perspective of 'why me?' but from a karmic viewpoint.

"As you know, there are two polarities of the self and the universe – Yin, the feminine principle, and Yang, the masculine principle. The feminine aspect is the feeling,

creative part of the self; the masculine deals with thought, the mind and acts of doing. Both polarities are manifested in humans at the physical level but, equally importantly, at the level of consciousness. Ultimately, we want to be in balance using both aspects.

"Whereas we as humans are a microcosm, the world is a macrocosm with the same structure. Looking at the structure of the universe in terms of feminine and masculine aspects, the Universe has the feminine at its center, the heart, using her intuitive feeling function to determine what must be created for the greatest good of all life. The feminine then engages the masculine energy to determine what actions need to take place to manifest this creation into being; thus, the Yin and Yang work in harmony. Unfortunately, our world has been completely out of balance for centuries, with the feminine aspect being denied and suppressed by the masculine principle.

"The male polarity has feared the feminine nature, with its unlimited creative power, judging it to be frightening, unsafe and unsure, because the Yin nature is associated with the unconscious, where all the mysteries of life spring forth. Manifesting things only through these fears, man desperately tries to deny, hide and control the feminine, in himself and in the world, so as not to unleash her unbounded power. The extreme physical manifestation of this need to control the feminine is the requirement of women to cover their entire bodies. On a global level, our world is on the brink of destruction due to all the male-driven economic corruption and warfare.

"The only solution to our predicament is to have the feminine lead us back to balance on both a microcosmic and macrocosmic level, with Mother Earth, the Divine

feminine archetype, leading the way. We as women can do our parts by placing the value on our feminine aspect that it deserves. This in turn will emanate outward into the world and help re-align the Universe so that it operates from its basic core – using its feminine nature to 'feel' what needs to be created, and then enlisting the masculine principle to 'manifest' its creation.

"*As for how this relates to my stroke, my masculine side (my right side) was completely paralyzed. Although we're talking about the physical body, psychologically speaking, I have always operated more out of my masculine side, being very controlling and aggressive, while suppressing much of my femininity (represented by the left side). The masculine had to be subdued if I ever wanted to achieve balance within.*

"*Thus my stroke...the Universe's way of helping me find this equilibrium between the masculine and feminine principles. I don't wish such trauma on anyone else seeking the same. This was my karma, and although I thought I had been working on balance for the past several years, I was still operating primarily from my masculine side, as what I was doing was more of an exercise of the mind (using control and force to make things happen) rather than of the heart (using intuition and feelings to guide my actions). As I recover, the process has moved from my head to my heart, where I am learning how to 'let go' and go with the flow of life, knowing I can't control everything that happens to me; and instead of being 'action-oriented' most of the time, I am now just 'being' with myself and allowing my creativity to flow.*

"*I must place more value on my feminine side so that I have an inner stasis, stability due to the harmony between the Yin and Yang within. As that occurs, my physical healing takes place while my feminine side takes over and helps bring my masculine side back to life. You've heard the saying 'Behind every good man, there's a good woman' and vice versa? Isn't that just another way of saying that Yin and Yang are balanced?"*

So what is my Truth as it relates to my stroke? How does it all tie together: my past-life experience and how it affected my current life, and the relationship between the masculine and feminine principles of our souls? And how will it help you in your own journey through your trauma? Let me boil it down to a few simple, easy-to-understand phrases.

Love and relationships are, in my mind, the basis of life; they go hand-in-hand. At the center are self-love and the inner relationship you have with yourself. If these two phenomena are strong, if you have found that balance within, you are living your life from your true essence, your authentic self. The stroke brought me home to my core essence. It made me realize my life circumstances did not define me; the stroke was not my life, but it helped me find that inner balance that made me whole. "Life is our deepest inner being [*not our outer presence*]. It is already whole, complete, perfect."⁴ It showed me that when you are whole within yourself, you are filled with pure love, and your outer relationships and circumstances are more meaningful because they become a reflection of your soul as it radiates that love. "...Only love is real.... Love never ends; it never stops. Its energy is absolute, eternal.... Love transcends everything else."⁵ Love knows no bounds. It knows no obstacles. It just is. And that's MY TRUTH!

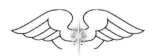

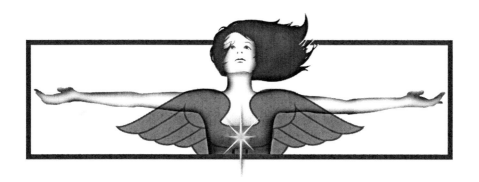

Never Give Up

"Never underestimate what you can achieve when you believe in yourself! Never, ever give up!"

A s I attempted to write this chapter, I was having great difficulty knowing what I wanted to say and how to say it. I had the concept in my mind and a story to tell, but the words didn't seem to want to flow like they did with my other three books. It wasn't writer's block as much as I was thinking and writing from a different perspective. I wasn't even able to elaborate on that because I didn't have the words to explain. It was just a very strong feeling inside that I had to go with. I thought that as I endeavored to write this chapter (and others), I would have more clarity, and maybe by the time I finished getting the words out, no matter how painful the process might be, I would have an explanation of why it was such a challenging journey writing this book, compared to my others.

The intro and first chapter of this book were relatively easy because I was telling my story, which I knew backwards and forwards; but as I wanted to provide insights on different topics, both spiritually and practically, the exercise of writing seemed a bit more arduous. I thought that maybe, just maybe, writing this chapter would help me ride this wave of uncertainty with the same determination I had to make a full recovery from my stroke. Isn't that what this chapter is all about? Facing our challenges with an interminable perseverance that you "never give up"?

I said in the introduction that I would be sharing stories of others who have also faced life-changing challenges and how they worked through them. The story I want to share now is of Deny, a man who embodies this passion, which helped him get through his trauma against all odds.

"At 20 years old, most of us are still in that 'invincible' state of mind. I was no different. On October 27, 1987, I was in my third year at the university and my doctor told me I had cancer. Which type of cancer? We didn't know yet. That would take another week or so. Once all of the poking, prodding and cutting were done, it turned out to be stage 2 Hodgkin's lymphoma. Believe it or not, it came as welcomed news. Of all of the possibilities, Hodgkin's disease was the most curable.

"By early November 1987, my parents and I sat down with my oncologist to determine the treatment plan. I was going to need six months of chemotherapy and eight weeks of radiation therapy. The good news, however, was that the prognosis was excellent – a 90% chance of being cured. So I resigned myself to the fact that I was going to have to put my life on hold for one year while they treated my cancer.

"In mid-August 1988, the long-awaited day finally came. Not only had I completed all my treatments, but I was also cancer-free! I didn't know it at the time, but it was only the very beginning of what was to be a most incredible journey.

"My cancer recurred in late October 1988. My cancer turned out to be more aggressive than the doctors

originally thought. It recurred again in early 1989, in the fall of 1990, the spring of 1991 and the summer of 2004. In all, I have fought cancer six times...despite being given a year to live after my recurrence in 1990.

"When you're fighting cancer, you go through a slew of emotions. Then come the side effects from the treatments: losing your hair, feeling nauseated all the time and general fatigue are only some of the physical challenges you face. Then, of course, there is the roller coaster of emotions. Very often, it feels like things are spiraling out of control. The biggest challenge is relinquishing that control and allowing yourself to heal. It seems rather counter-intuitive to do so, but it is necessary. Knowing when to relinquish control and when to take it back is THE BIGGEST challenge that took me 16 years of living with cancer to overcome. Ironically, it is also what saved my life.

"Between 1987 and 1991, not one year went by when I wasn't fighting cancer in one way or another. One can just imagine the toll this can take on a person. I have to admit, while there were many good and even wonderful times during that period of my life, there were also many very bad times.

"I was blessed to have had faith in our Creator from a very early age. This faith got me through many a bad time when all seemed hopeless. Nevertheless, I kept moving forward with faith that everything that was happening to me was for a reason I have yet to know. I looked at my cancer journey as a series of finish lines I needed to cross in order to complete the race. Every time I started a chemotherapy treatment, I would tell myself, 'Just get through the next 12 hours and all will be okay.' Every time my cancer came back, I would tell myself,

'Okay, just get through these next few months and all will be fine.' I had to do that over and over again. Giving up was not an option. In my book Many Shades of Green – Running Toward the Finish Line, One Cancer at a Time, *I wrote: 'Survivors never complain or dwell on their current situation. Instead they move forward with an ever-present focus on the horizon.' It was my faith, however, that gave me the strength to keep my focus and cross the next 'finish line'.*

"I have been cancer-free since 2004. When I look back on my journey, I can honestly say cancer was the best thing that has ever happened to me. You should see the look I get from people when I tell them that. However, it is true. I would not be the person I am today, were it not for cancer. Through all my pain and suffering, I became the person I was meant to become, as opposed to the person I thought I was supposed to be. I received enlightenment beyond any level I could ever imagine. I realized that being well didn't just mean healing my body; it meant healing my mind and my spirit, as well. For if one of these elements suffers, they all suffer.

"Today, I have a beautiful life. I still have physical and emotional scars that stem from the cancer treatments, but most of them are healing. I think I will always have some scars to remind me of what I have been through, but that's okay. I have 'made friends' with them. This may sound strange to some people, but part of the healing process includes accepting and loving myself, including my cancer. Although my cancer did not define me as a person, it was part of me, and if I was to love myself, I had to love my cancer as well. Love, you see, is the greatest healing power of all.

"From 1991 to 2004 (between my fifth and sixth bouts), I had a 13-year break from cancer. Just before my last recurrence, however, God sent me an angel (my wife Theresa) to make certain I got through it safe and sound. Thanks to her kindness and tenacity, not only did I get through it, but together we found ways to achieve wellness on all three levels: body, mind and spirit. Thanks to her, I am completely alive!"

As Deny's story illustrates, you should never, ever give up. Never underestimate what you can achieve when you believe in yourself, knowing that you have a very special purpose in life.

When I first started writing this book, I wasn't fully recovered, but I knew I would be. I had faith! Oh, there were good days and bad days. I regressed sometimes, and when I did, I felt like I would be as I was for the rest of my life. But I kept working physically, emotionally and spiritually on my recovery. Physically, between rehab and my home exercise program, I worked out five times a week. Emotionally and spiritually, I knew part of my healing was to stop trying to control everything, "to surrender and let go," just as Deny said.

Remember that I had always been controlled by the masculine element of my psyche, with its need to dominate its surroundings. In order to find the inner balance between the masculine and feminine aspects within my psyche, I needed to relinquish my need to control everything and become more passive, knowing I could surrender to Spirit, the co-creator of my life. I didn't have the last say in my recovery, since Spirit has ultimate power over our lives, but I believed that I would heal, even though it wouldn't be by my timeline. I did my part in my healing, as I was very diligent about my rehab and exercise. But then I turned it over to the Higher Power and let Spirit do the rest.

When you believe in yourself, you send the energy of that belief out into the Universe, which sets things in motion. Upon hearing your belief or request, Spirit will then provide you with whatever resources you need to honor that belief – the right doctors; the right therapists, be they psychological or physical; the right procedures and techniques; the right people to support you, be they family and friends or those who simply cross your path at just the right moment for whatever it is they are to offer you as you travel the road to redemption. "Ask and ye shall receive!"

Remember at the beginning of the chapter I told you I had no explanation for why this book was so challenging for me? Well, I had an epiphany as I was "chatting" on Facebook with a book-writing group, a group of folks with whom I was taking an online book-writing class. Here is what I said.

"I have been pondering why I'm having so much more trouble writing this book than I did with my other books, but I think I figured it out! :-) I was much, much more organized and structured with my other books. I had a plan. With this one, I have little organization. But that's okay, because I'm writing this one from a very different perspective. Let's just say I'm shifting from operating out of my masculine side (with its order and need to control) to creating from my feminine side (where creativity is born).

"You see, I've lived my life (pre-stroke) being dictated by the male aspect of my psyche. My feminine side didn't have a chance. My stroke has turned this around. The right side of my body (representing the masculine) was the side that was paralyzed. Well, it had to die in a sense (or should I say, lose control) so that my left side could take over and come into its full power. (Isn't that what's happening in the world? The Divine Feminine is coming back into power to balance the masculine?) Thus,

it has also manifested in the way I am writing my book. Does this all make sense? It's pretty exciting to me to see how my book is such a significant part of my healing. Woohoo!"

This is my Truth and this book is part of that truth. It's serving its purpose in my healing. I could not continue operating as before. My mind had no plan of what I was going to write about. This was such an emotional journey that it was hard to put order into telling the story. I would write whatever moved inside me. I couldn't follow an outline. It would have taken away the heart-based tone. It was a lesson that I was to learn about surrendering – to move from ego-consciousness to heart-consciousness, going from thinking from "with-OUT," where organization was the order of the day, to thinking from "within," where creativity is sparked – moving from the masculine to the feminine.

My mind was like a kaleidoscope of thoughts, each wanting to talk at the same time, with no rhyme or reason. Maybe it was an effect of the stroke...the disorientation, the lack of focus...maybe it was a cognitive dysfunction. But I would have none of that thinking! So, you know what I did? I surrendered. I let go and turned it over to Spirit. I asked for guidance and I received it. I became a passive vessel through which the Higher Power worked. I knew I was in communion with the source of creativity and I let it have its way with me. I didn't fight my mind; struggling was senseless. It would only paralyze me so that I couldn't write at all. I wrote passages that I would eventually weave into the chapters of this book where they were best suited. My mind jumped from one thought to the next and as it did, I would just write down what it was regurgitating.

What does this have to do with the theme of this chapter: "never give up"? With my revelation about writing from a different perspective, I gained the clarity I needed to understand why I felt so challenged in writing this book. I'm sure you've often heard "knowledge is power." By receiving the insights of what made me feel "stuck" in the throes of my uncertainty, I felt empowered as the Divine Feminine moved through me, helping me to create. I hadn't given up in my ongoing quest for my Truth, in all its various scenarios. I believed I could find the way. I believed in myself! And I NEVER gave up!

So I ask of you: what are you going to do? You have experienced tragedy in your life. It has incapacitated you in some way. Are you going to let it make you or break you? Do you have the wherewithal to challenge yourself to the nth degree? No matter what, no matter how many falls you take, get right back up, dust yourself off and stand tall in your beliefs, in yourself and in Spirit, your co-creator. Nothing is more powerful than the human spirit when it is guided by the Divine Spirit. With Spirit at the helm, you can achieve anything!

EXERCISE

Get out your journal (or notebook) and write down positive affirmations that you can say to yourself when you feel you want to give up. Then, any time you're at an emotional low and you want to hang it all up, recite some of your affirmations quietly or out loud. If need be, shout your affirmations for emphasis, knowing that the Universe hears you no matter how loudly you repeat the words and it will support you. Words have powerful energy and sending your message out into the Universe can have a strong impact on how you feel. One of my favorites is, *"The power that created my body heals my body."*

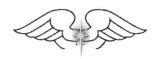

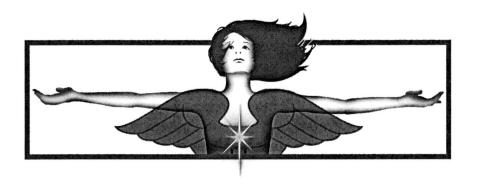

You Knew Your Trauma
before You Were Born

"Because of the sacred contracts we have made with the Divine, we are given the opportunity to come into our personal power. When we reach this majestic realm of elevated consciousness, we experience 'heaven on earth' – and isn't that a great place to be?"

Did you know that before we are born, we make a pact with the Divine as to what kind of life we will have, e.g. who our parents are going to be, what life situations we will encounter, what relationships we will be in? This "sacred contract" is the means by which you are given the chance to awaken your Divine potential, making the best use of your personal power throughout your life. "Think of your sacred contract as a life course in which you are meant to learn many lessons!"[6] You must discover what you are meant to do in your life and the Divine promises to provide the guidance you need to fulfill your obligations. This can mean being guided into certain relationships or developing an illness, among other ways, good and bad.

There are five stages one goes through when following one's sacred contract: contact, heeding the call, renaming, assignments and surrender. As all the stages overlap and interweave throughout your life, you may go through them more than once in your life as the challenges or circumstances change in your life. First, you make a connection with the Divine in some way, whether through "ordinary" or "extraordinary" circumstances, such as through dreams, meditation or some serendipitous event such as my stroke. Once you've made this connection, it's up to you to take action on what this experience has awakened in you. This is usually when you see life from a different perspective and with a whole new set of values, with the desire to serve others. By embarking on your path, you may take on a new name or a new role that has more spiritual meaning. You may create a sacred space at home, start meditating, create a spiritual community, work with a spiritual teacher, etc. You will be faced with challenges that are in fact opportunities to help you continue down your path of growth. These life-changing moments will likely go against the grain, impelling you to make changes you may not have otherwise made. To fulfill your contract, it will be crucial that you surrender to the will of the Divine, which will push you further and further down the path of your spiritual development.

To assist you in attaining this higher purpose of your life, there are inner forces that are directly involved in the day-to-day structure of your life – how you live, whom you love, why certain relationships have been necessary and why you have had to take on certain tasks that may have been burdensome and destructive. They help you learn to understand yourself on a very profound level, realizing that everything has its role in your life, regardless of how painful or joyful it may be. No one is in your life by accident – not your parents, not your friends or family, nor your adversaries. And no circumstance you encounter is a coincidence. By agreeing to your sacred contract, you agree to learn lessons throughout your time as a living, breathing earthly being. These dynamic inner energies are archetypal patterns commonly found in many people's emotions and thoughts, across cultures and countries. They are the architects of your life, the governing forces of your psyche and soul. They connect you to your sacred contract – to your greater mission on Earth.

According to Caroline Myss, author of *Sacred Contracts*, there are four universal archetypal patterns that work through all people's lives: the Child, the Victim, the Prostitute and the Saboteur. They are the four archetypes of "survival," symbolizing our major life challenges and how we choose to survive. Myss says it like this:

> "These four archetypes are like the four legs of a table on which our sacred contract rests.... They need to be stable to support the weight of the tabletop – our life mission.... They make you conscious of your vulnerabilities, your fear of being victimized. They allow you to see how you sabotage your creative opportunities or abort your dreams, and in the future will become your allies in fulfilling opportunities and dreams. Your archetypes...will preserve your integrity, refusing to allow you to negotiate it away under any circumstance."[7]

The following story illustrates how the Child archetype, with its many aspects – the Innocent Child, the Wounded Child, the Abandoned or Orphaned Child, the Dependent Child, the Nature Child and the Divine Child – had a profound impact on Aurelio, a man whose childhood trauma continued to haunt him in his marital relationship. The Child's attention is on the awareness of life, safety, nurturing, loyalty and family, with its core issues being dependency and responsibility. If we have ideally matured through the stages of growing up (from the utter dependency as a child to being a self-conscious, self-centered adolescent, to our teens when we first become aware of our vulnerabilities as well as our strengths and talents, to the transition into a responsible

31

adult), then there will likely be little dysfunction in our ability to be responsible, independent individuals in our relationships and our endeavors. However, "when these cycles are not followed in some way, adults will find it difficult if not impossible to be responsible for themselves in the physical world and to create successful relationships."[8] Here is Aurelio's story:

"The trauma started as a young boy. It was the emotional abuse from my parents, especially my mother...yelling at me constantly...saying the worst things you could possibly say to a human being: 'I WISH SOMEONE WOULD KILL YOU!! I WISH SOMEONE WOULD POISON YOU!! I WISH YOU WOULD GET CANCER!!'

"That is just a taste of what I experienced every day, every week, every year, growing up as a first-generation Italian-Canadian. The words my mother screamed at me would cut to my very soul. I didn't know why she said those things to me; I just knew that she did. Those words. That energy. That loudness. It hurt my ears. And it killed a part of me deep within.

"I didn't know it at the time, but I had suppressed all the hurt and tormented feelings I had of being abandoned, abused, and mistreated. Growing up, I felt like I was totally worthless. That there must be something very wrong with me...something very bad and broken about me. That my own parents could say such unspeakable things to me...with such conviction and such force...day after day...year after year...that it must be true.

"Such feelings continued through my marriage, and I came to realize afterwards that I used my marriage to replay my emotionally troubled childhood. I would project my mother onto my wife and try to seek revenge

through her for the hurts my mother perpetrated on me. I would customize the criticisms I received from my mother and throw them onto my wife."

How could a mom be so abusive to her own flesh and blood? To a child who depended on her for his physical and psychological wellbeing? Wasn't she supposed to nurture him, love and care for him to ensure that he blossomed into a fine, independent, responsible man who could fearlessly conquer his own world? But apparently, her abuse was part of the sacred contract Aurelio made with his mother before he was born. And instead of being the Innocent Child safely protected in a loving environment, Aurelio's Wounded Child spent years trying to heal and compensate for the deficiencies of his formative years in life. This was felt primarily through the troubled relationship he had with his wife, which ended in a painful divorce.[9]

However, by connecting with his Innocent Child in the later years of his life, he was able to restore his life. The Innocent Child helps heal and stop the abuse of the Wounded Child, inspiring one to appreciate oneself by initiating a new relationship or creative endeavor – whatever it takes to feel nurtured or cared for. Aurelio found solace in tears and music to heal his wounded psyche.

"I cried a lot...and wrote songs to express all that was within me. And at the end of the crying sessions, I would feel a taste of inner peace...which allowed me to go forward for the hour or day."

Two sides of his inner child had come out to play (pardon the pun!), to reveal one of the lessons he needed to learn – self-love – and to help him work through the hurt and pain inflicted on him at such a young age, so that he could learn to love himself and thrive.

"Through years of therapy, counseling and intense personal work on myself, I've worked through those powerful emotions and ignored feelings to heal those parts of myself, and to have a much healthier and more loving relationship with my mother and my deceased father. I can now see how much they did love me, but because of their own issues and limitations, they were unable to express that love in a way that I could appreciate."

As he gained spiritual insight into his situation, Aurelio was able to transform his life from one of merely surviving (*"Fear of doing anything...fear of taking care of myself, feeding myself, etc. – irrational fears, yet very real to me"*) to one of compassion and love. (*"I have a 'higher level' view of the situation.... I love my mother and deceased father more than ever before, and I can appreciate them much more for the gifts they gave me and continue to give me."*)

I used only one archetype in describing Aurelio's situation for the sake of simplicity, and because it was the most applicable to the circumstances. As the guardian of innocence, the Child archetype was the energy pattern that revealed itself to protect Aurelio's innocence, to protect him from the pain and suffering he experienced at the hands of his mother, and to help him reclaim his life. It came forth in different forms throughout his life when the need arose, first as the Wounded Child and then as the Innocent Child.

In addition to the four survival archetypes – Child, Victim, Saboteur and Prostitute – other archetypes that come forth depending on our life circumstances include the Matriarch (or Mother), Patriarch (or Father), Queen, King, Goddess/God, Warrior, Slave, Steward, Messenger, Rebel, Muse, Martyr, Hermit, Mystic, Visionary and Healer, just to name a few (for more, see appendix in *Sacred Contracts*). We must delve into our psyches to find the ones that have been most prevalent in our lives, to see what has conditioned our behavior, thoughts and actions.

In addition to the many archetypal patterns that dictate how we behave, there is another concept that plays a big role in the choices we make in fulfilling our sacred contract: the Shadow, the so-called "dark side" of our psyche, "the negative side of the personality, the sum of all unpleasant qualities [one likes] to hide..."[10], the realm in which our fears dance. Let me use my own story to demonstrate how the Shadow plays its part on the stage of our life. It can be your ally or it can be your opponent, depending on how you relate to it. Note that all archetypes, being part of your psyche, have their shadow side.

The Saboteur archetypal pattern, as one of my Shadow figures, showed its face throughout my life, treading over my self-esteem time and time again. Despite all I did in my life – being a ballet dancer and pianist, a first degree black belt in Tae Kwon Do, author, Reiki master, massage therapist, life coach, and corporate manager at a Fortune 500 company, in addition to being a wife for 16 1/2 years and a mother of 2 wonderful young men – I never thought I was good enough. Maybe that's why I did so much...to prove that I could be something. But for everything I did, I never fully followed through with any of them, except for being a mom, which is innate in women and governed by the Matriarch/Mother archetype.

The Saboteur used its power to crush any efforts in happiness and success, no matter what I did. It all culminated when I began my foray into entrepreneurship. It seemed I could never get my endeavors to a point where they could sustain me financially and emotionally. Deep inside, the Saboteur was putting up all the road blocks that prevented me from reaching that place of inner peace and security (where my fears of being successful would dissipate, instead of treading all over my soul) and the manifested outer reality of financial stability.

Then I had my stroke, which changed everything. The shadow side of the Saboteur was no longer in power. Three months after my stroke, I had a series of serious anxiety attacks. Each morning, I would wake up in a state of terror that lasted all day unless I took medication, which I rarely did since it was addictive. I suffered terribly during that period, with thoughts of suicide dancing through my head.

Fortunately, they finally subsided after about a month. When I turned inward to try to find an answer to the madness, I learned that it was actually a purging of all my fears that had accumulated throughout my life. They had come on with such fury that I thought I would go insane. But as they bubbled up from the dark crevices of my psyche and arose into the "light," I was released from the claws of my archetypal foe. I had confronted the Shadow side of my Saboteur archetype and had been victorious in quelling its power over me. The Saboteur was now my friend, my companion. By pouncing on my soul, trying to make me feel I wasn't good enough to accomplish anything, it allowed me to bring its actions (disguised as anxieties) into the light of consciousness. By eclipsing my fears, I was able to give birth to my personal power. So as I continued with my recovery, I was in the gestation phase of my resurrection, my awakening of fresh opportunities that awaited me. I *would* reach my divine potential, fulfilling my sacred contract.

We grow through the relationships and challenges presented to us in our lives, leading us down the path to that intimate place where our soul communes with the omnipotent, omniscient Source of all life. Because of the sacred contracts we have made with the Divine, we are given the opportunity to come into our personal power. When we reach this majestic realm of elevated consciousness, we experience "heaven on earth" – and isn't that a great place to be?

NOTE: I only scratched the surface of the topic of sacred contracts. My goal was for you to realize how your life trauma is a glorious treasure, a gift from the heavens, no matter how daunting it is. It changes your view of life. It helps you see who you really are – the celestial being that you are, from whom the sparks of the Divine radiate.

EXERCISE

(You may need to get Caroline Myss' book *Sacred Contracts* to do this exercise, or borrow it from your local library.) Get out your journal or notebook. Determine one archetype that has come into play in your life. Does it relate to your trauma and how you're coping with the circumstance? If so, how? If not, how has it affected you in some other aspect of your life?

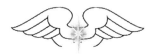

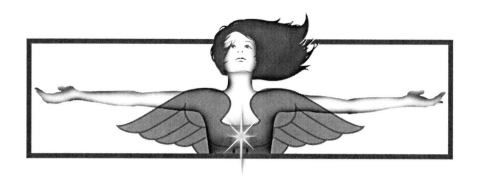

Limiting Beliefs:
What You Believe, You Receive

> *"The more we focus on our limiting beliefs, the more powerful they become.... You can reprogram your limiting beliefs of the past to something more positive and nurturing."*

I was on my way to rehab on a wonderfully brisk day (Houston was finally being wrapped in the arms of autumn, even though it was already almost Thanksgiving) and I made a discovery that was born out of a feeling I'd had a few days before. I had been faced with the fear that I wouldn't fully recover, which sent me into a tailspin of despondency. Would I be able to walk normally again? Would I be able to return to my salsa dance lessons? Would my arm ever have all of its strength back, or would it always feel like a dissociated appendage? Would I ever have the energy to get back to my business – my Reiki and massage, my books, my life coaching? Could I still be a good mom to my boys? Would I be able to reconnect with the love of my life?

For a few days, that fear kept rolling around in my head like a bowling ball, with me as its target. I was a lone bowling pin, unstable and wavering, waiting to be knocked down into the chute, only to be lifted up again, to be knocked down again...and again...and again. Would I ever be able to escape that loop of constant "mind chatter" that fed my fear? Never mind that I had just written the chapter "Never Give Up!" or that I always tried to remind myself to "surrender and let go," to release my fears to the Universe. Never mind that I had received countless inner messages that I would fully recover. My body didn't seem to be progressing; in fact, I felt like I was regressing, at times.

But then I had my revelation, and it was this: I was actually preventing my full recovery because of my "limiting beliefs." Can you believe that? Me, who couldn't wait to recover so I could get on with my life. Me, who had so much to do, so many plans that didn't include being sick for the rest of my life or even another few months. So where were these fears coming from? What did this resistance to my healing represent?

While I pondered these questions, my first thought was that by recovering, I would have to be independent and responsible again, and although I desperately wanted that, it was a scary prospect since for the past year-and-a-half, I'd been relying on my mom for support. But then an image came to mind, of a recurring dream I used to have, and I felt it had everything to do with my fear.

I was on a 3x3 platform, high, high above a body of water...a large lake...the ocean...I wasn't sure. All I knew was that I was petrified of falling. I was so high in the sky. THE SKY! In mythological or religious contexts, the sky is associated with the masculine principle – as the heavenly Father, or Zeus/Jupiter as the God over the heavens, or Apollo as the Sun God. Native Americans hold reverent Father Sky in creation myths. In Ancient Egypt, Horus is the ruler of the sky. In China, Tian (meaning sky or heavens) is one of the oldest terms for the cosmos and a key concept in Chinese mythology and religion, relating to the masculine element.

Another view of Father Sky is that the principle is associated with the right side of the body, which is the analytical, masculine side. And of course, it goes without saying, then, that Mother Earth would be associated with the left side, the feminine side. Sound familiar? As Carl G. Jung said, "Heaven is masculine, but earth is feminine. Therefore, God has his throne in heaven while Wisdom has hers on the earth."[11]

Mother Earth represents one's nurturing side, housing the creative force. Ideas that manifest in material form in outer reality are all seeds within the inner realm of spiritual and mental creation – that is, the feminine unconscious part of your psyche, where intuition sparks. Within this domain of the "great mysteries of life," all things exist. It can be likened to the ocean, the Great Ocean of our subconscious. Looking at the ocean, we only see the surface. But below are the great mysteries and unknowns. The deep recesses of the ocean represent the deep recesses of our subconscious, which exist in their un-manifested forms, waiting to be discovered so they can become reality – our Truths.

So why was I so fearful of falling into the waters of the unconscious, to activate my feminine side? After all, I am female! But as you know from my story, I'd been basking in the sun's rays of the masculine for a long time and I guess I became very comfortable in that high position where I could exert power, authority and dominion over my life. I was ambitious, analytical and aggressive, and I had a strong will. I was emotionally distant, somewhat aloof, and I had trouble getting too intimate with people because my heart was closed. To fall into the water, where emotions and intuition reign, and where I had no control due the "unknowingness" of what could bubble up to the surface – wouldn't that leap have been a plunge to a death of sorts? To be thrust out of my comfort zone where I could direct all aspects of my life, into a place where I was no longer in the driver's seat?

I began to see how this dream, though from the past, had such significance in my current circumstances. I made the association of taking the plunge into the depths as a means for me to find that balance between the masculine and feminine, to "becom[e] whole within myself" as I said in "My Story." By becoming whole and thus speaking with my authentic voice, I COULD direct my life, but from a very different standpoint. Instead of living my life from "without," as I always had, from the outer reality of the tangible physical world, where the masculine rules, I could live my life from "within," from my feminine essence where creativity and intuition radiate outward, and where self-love is born. And from this place of pure love, I could reach out to others with that same love. My stroke was a way to open my heart, allowing the Divine presence within to permeate my life and surround others with its warm glow of love and compassion.

So into the depths of the Great Ocean I had fallen. I decided then that I wasn't going to let my limiting beliefs overcome me. I have a purpose in life, as we all do. As I continued my recovery, I wished to help others in their recovery from their calamities – to show them the treasures they are receiving from their experience, and how destructive their limiting beliefs can be in realizing these gifts. They can prevent you from reaching your highest potential, from realizing your mission on Earth. Your life loses its richness because you aren't able to perceive it correctly. You begin to see life through the filters of these beliefs, which are a result of words, thoughts and experiences that you internalize as your Truths – telling you that you aren't good enough or worthy, or that you don't deserve anything, or that you aren't lovable or you are incapable of loving. According to Don Miguel Ruiz, Toltec Shaman and author of *The Four Agreements*, "You see everything is about belief. What we believe rules our existence, rules our life."

Pamina's story below shows how these false truths that we internalize can ravage our lives until we extinguish their hold on us and replace them with ones that empower us instead.

"You want to be what? Don't be stupid! What does a girl need qualifications for? I'm not wasting money on your education," my father announced. Predictably this post-hypnotic suggestion took root – and I used it as an excuse for nonperformance, for years. I had given all my power away and had no vision of who I was, where I wanted to be or why. So through default, I teetered on the edge of disaster, again and again. Procrastination paralysis became my way of ensuring that if I never actually did it (whatever it was I was procrastinating about), I couldn't fail – or succeed. I was waging a full-scale war against myself. My insecurities were visible from the next solar system – without a telescope. No matter how fast I ran or where I tried to hide, my own fears kept ambushing me.

"I had also developed SRS (Serial Rescuing Syndrome), consistently getting caught in a debilitating cycle of need dependency, frequently forming attachments to people who sucked the life force out of me. I relinquished all power in my life.

"Then at 29, I inflicted this powerless person on (you guessed it!) an equally powerless man. We got married and I fell pregnant with my first child. I didn't know it then, but my life was about to rival the Dakar Rally as an endurance test. When I look back, I think, 'Imagine inflicting a legacy like that on a child!' But this was no ordinary child. 'Your baby is a mongol. She has a heart abnormality and won't live long. She'll never walk, talk or feed herself. I advise you to put her in a home and

forget about her,' were the devastating words of the pediatrician.

"The term 'emotional meltdown' doesn't begin to cover it. But amid this unimaginable turmoil, I was handed a lifebelt – Louise Hay's You Can Heal Your Life *– and a splinter of Louise's spirit slipped silently between my heartbeats, where it took up permanent residence. In time, we became inseparable companions on a rollercoaster sojourn of self-discovery. My deeply entrenched disdain for authority figures served me well during this time. 'Can't, won't, hasn't and will-never-be' poured forth from many learned lips over the years. And so the inside-out game was born. Every 'can't' became a 'can' and every 'won't' became a 'will.' After a while it became downright addictive; 'Great! We have a problem – let's turn it inside-out!'*

"My diminutive, damaged angel survived for 16 years and, fortunately, during the course of those 16 years, my anger found a million opportunities to burn itself out, as it gave me the impetus to demolish obstacle after obstacle, with its righteous rage. I vented my frustration on doctors whose ignorance was only superseded by their arrogant conviction that there was no such term as Down's syndrome; educationists whose tunnel vision or self-serving goals pronounced Michelle (my daughter) uneducable; and [I endured] nauseatingly opinionated people who had all the answers to a challenge they had never faced.

"The force of my anger gave me the strength to insist that Michelle not be swept under the carpet and ignored or conveniently sidelined, and in my role of Warrior Mom, I grew braver and more fearless by the day. My marriage, though, caught in the whiplash of this

whirlwind, ripped at the seams. The life blood leaked from it at a perilous rate.

"The only way out of the mess, I ultimately learned, was to begin the kind of love affair I dreamed about, with myself. I learned to be my own cheerleader, celebrating each and every triumph – and the momentum built daily. And once I realized it was me who created my bliss or my mess, I took a deep breath, plucked up the courage to squint through some pretty powerful binoculars and performed a ruthless autopsy on my relating skills. Not pretty. Nobody else to blame for the havoc I had created. No excuses or justifications to hide behind. I started to make myself loveable!"

Overcoming limiting beliefs takes some work. It can be a lifelong process, depending upon how deep these beliefs are and how much they have pervaded your psyche. Remember, the Shadow side of your psyche, which can dictate limiting beliefs, can have long destructive tentacles, which wrap around your mind and make you believe the worst about yourself. In *My Stroke of Insight*, Dr. Jill Bolte Taylor, a Harvard-trained brain scientist who had a massive hemorraghic stroke at 37 years old, leaving her unable to walk, talk, read, write, or recall any of her life, explains scientifically how our brains process the information we take in. "The more conscious attention we pay to any particular circuit, or the more time we spend thinking specific thoughts, the more impetus those circuits or thought patterns have to run again with minimal external stimulation."[12] In other words, the more we focus on our limiting beliefs, the more powerful they become.

"At some point in the growing up process, many of us are programmed to believe that challenges are problems; that problems are bad; something to dread, avoid or sink

into an abyss of despair about; something to be rescued from or medicate ourselves into avoiding. But by doing this we're missing the plot completely. Suffering the consequences of our actions is the only way we mature, and what we learn from these experiences benefits others who are struggling with similar challenges. Instead of being an indelible mark of shame, every mess I make and overcome empowers me to help others who are making similar messes. Accepting challenges has the potential to grant me grace.... I learned not to underestimate the power of our parental relating patterns; how deeply they are imprinted in our psyches.

"Just as feeling the sting of rejection is a certainty in life, every one of us has experienced being dumped by a partner, losing a job, not being chosen for the team, being fired or retrenched, being betrayed, ridiculed, diminished or performing below expectation. But people's careless comments, expectations, aborted dreams, fears, personal agendas or perceptions of reality no longer have a profound effect on the choices I make. It's only an opinion. I refuse to allow rejection to cripple or define me."

As Dr. Taylor, who spent eight years of persistent work fully recovering from her stroke, points out, "Our left hemisphere thinks in patterned responses to incoming stimulation. It establishes neurological circuits that run relatively automatically to sensory information.... [It] creates...'loops of thought patterns' [and] is superb at predicting what we will think, how we will act, or what we will feel in the future – based on our past experiences."[13] As our left mind governs the right side of our body, the masculine side, it creates our limiting beliefs, through critical judgment and analysis. And the right mind, which governs the left or feminine side of the body, is the well from which compassion, self-love and creativity spring forth.

"[The] right mind is open to new possibilities and thinks out of the box. It is not limited to the rules and regulations established by [the] left mind that created that box.... [It] brings new insights...so [you] can update old files that contain outdated information."[14] In other words, by shifting the control of the inner masculine critic to the power of the inner feminine divinity, you can reprogram your limiting beliefs of the past to something more positive and nurturing.

"When I rewind the movie of this tumultuous and eventful time, it's the difficult times that are most memorable; that contained the seeds of my most powerful revelations...the choice of whether to let [them] cripple or empower me is always mine.

"I have learned to embrace change and live in the moment; to be flexible and adapt to a variety of environments and circumstances. Having gained first-hand experience of how quickly and unexpectedly those you love can disappear from your life has increased the intensity of my love and appreciation; granted me the ability to instantly discern between a looming crisis and a blip on the radar screen.

"I know what it feels like to be in a 'less resourceful state.' It used to be my default program – and it sucks! Now, I just take a deep breath, press the pause button and use the following criteria: Does this reaction empower or disempower me? It really is that simple; and the choice I make determines the outcome."

I previously mentioned how I wasn't going to let my limiting beliefs overcome me – and I'm not! And yet as I continued writing this chapter, they had taken hold of me (only slightly, though!). I was talking to my mom, telling her I

47

needed to regain strength in my arm and get rid of the stiffness in my hand. I remembered that my occupational therapist said her goal was to get me functionally recovered so I could return to my world of service to others. Well, since I'm a massage therapist, didn't it make sense that starting to give massages again would help the strength and stiffness of my arm and hand, preparing me for my full re-entry into that world?

My mom thought it to be a grand idea, especially since she would be one of my guinea pigs for regular daily massages (who wouldn't think of it as a grand idea if they were getting regular massages). Then that little inner voice from the past spoke to me. "You won't be able to do it. You've never had much stamina. You'll get too tired. You don't have enough strength." I immediately said to my mom that I would only be able to give five-minute massages, since that was all my arm and hand could handle. She snapped back at me (kindly, of course!) and reminded me that I was letting my limiting beliefs hinder me. Why should I set a "limit" on how long I could give a massage before I even tried giving one? So, without further ado, I gave Mom her first massage, doing as much as I could. And at every occupational or physical therapy session I went to thereafter, I gave at least one therapist a massage, allowing me to regain the strength in my arm and reduce the stiffness in my hand. The question now was, "Who is the patient: the therapist or me?" That little inner voice couldn't tread over my soul any longer. I had dethroned it.

The plasticity of the brain – its ability to repair, replace and retrain its neural circuitry – allows us to change our limiting beliefs. "With focused attention...you can change your thoughts, change your activities, and change your behaviors to make a positive improvement in your life...stop feeding the old circuitry that reinforces your fears and anger and, instead, direct your attention toward new, positive neural connections."[15]

As this chapter came to a close, I realized I was truly beginning to integrate the male and female aspects of my psyche – that inner divinity and the embodiment of my life in outer reality. I was becoming whole. After I wrote down my thoughts in a less-than-organized (OK, chaotic!) form, just trying to let the ideas from the creative realm inside flow, the masculine taskmaster took over and put order into those thoughts so they made sense. And my original fear of having to be independent and responsible again no longer existed. My limiting beliefs were fading away. The feminine and masculine were working in concert, making beautiful music together. I was on my way to full recovery – physically, mentally, emotionally and spiritually!

EXERCISE

Get out your journal or notebook and write down all your limiting beliefs in the left column and what positive thoughts and behaviors you can embrace to change them in the right column. If at any time your mind starts to chatter, repeating your limiting beliefs, call for your empowering inner voice to repeat the positive thoughts instead. Likewise, use one of the positive behaviors you have listed to help snuff out the negativity of your thoughts.

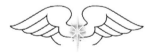

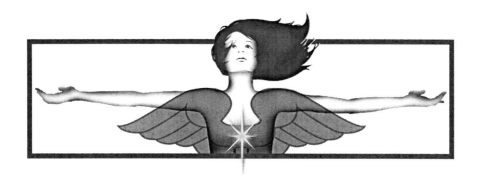

Gratitude and Attitude

"Gratitude and attitude have everything to do with how a person will travel through the treacherous waters of adversity.... A positive attitude brings optimism into your life, even in the direst situations.... If you adopt it as a way of life, great things can come your way."

It was a month before Christmas and my last day at rehab for the year. My sessions for the year had ended, so for the month of December, I would just do my home exercise program and go to the gym until the New Year started and sessions resumed.

As I worked with my physical therapist, I started reminiscing about when I first had my stroke a year-and-a-half before. Since the therapist was fairly new at the center, she hadn't been with me from the beginning. I related to her how I had been wheelchair-bound and I couldn't even lift a finger. Now I was walking (even jogging some) and had use of my arm and hand. I had come a long way, baby! I still had a way to go, but I was on my path to full recovery. She was shocked that I had done so well in such a short time. Now to me, a-year-and-a-half was like "forever," but considering the context of what I'd been through, she said I had made phenomenal progress. It could have taken years to recover, as it did for Dr. Taylor, mentioned in the previous chapter. It took her eight years to recover fully.

Every stroke is unique and affects each person differently. Dr. Taylor had a hemorraghic stroke that flooded her brain with blood, wiping out all her cognitive abilities, as well as disabling her physically. I had an ischemic stroke caused by a blood clot, and because I received the appropriate medicine (the "clot blaster" as they called the tPA) in time, my stroke really only affected my motor skills. Yes, it did have some residual effects on my speech and my ability to think clearly and process information, but for the most part, all I had was hemiplegia (paralysis of one side of the body). If I hadn't received the medicine so soon, my stroke would have been much more profound, potentially as serious as Dr. Taylor's, or maybe even worse.

From the day I had my stroke, Spirit was there with me every step of the way, guiding everything perfectly so that I had the best doctors, the best therapists, the best medical support and support from family and friends. Even my insurance coverage proved to be fabulous, so I wasn't burdened with financial woes. Oh, there were some minor snafus, like when one of my nurses wasn't careful and let me fall. I also found out who my real friends were. The person I thought was my best friend didn't come to see me even once at the hospital when I first had my stroke. Her excuse was that she had her own problems to contend with. As I saw it, we all have problems in some fashion. If we waited until we had no problems at all before we helped someone else, we would never get around to reaching out to others. Isn't that a little self-centered? Aren't we supposed to help our fellow man (or woman, as the case may be)? It took me awhile to get over her behavior, since she had been a best friend for years, but I finally shifted my feelings from resentment and hurt to acceptance. I couldn't control her actions, but I could control my response.

And as I continued to move up the path of recovery, I looked back and saw all I had learned. I am so grateful for the blessings I've received by having a stroke. I know that sounds crazy but I have much to be thankful for. "Gratitude unlocks the fullness of life. It turns what we have into enough, and more. It turns denial into acceptance, chaos into order, confusion to clarity."[16] My stroke showed me how resilient I am. Being debilitated gave me time to re-evaluate my life and recognize what's really important in life. It taught me patience and how to let go and surrender. It showed me that I don't have to live my life alone, that I am supported and protected by the co-creator of my life, the Divine. It gave new meaning to my life, helping me fulfill my destiny of helping others.

It allowed me to write this book, which I wish to be an inspiration to others in their time of need. It moved me into the present moment, instead of dwelling on the past or worrying about the future. It helped me overcome many of the anxieties I had lived with all my life. It changed my perspective in life, moving me from an ego-based consciousness to a heart-based consciousness. It taught me that faith goes a long way to manifest positivity in our lives. It revealed to me that our life situation is not who we are. And finally, I made some wonderful friendships with people from all over the world during my journey. One such friend's story is as follows.

Gratitude and attitude have everything to do with how a person will travel through the treacherous waters of adversity, as Callie's journey to becoming a breast cancer warrior goddess reveals:

"In 2011 BC (before cancer!), I was toddling along in life. My son, my only child, had left home to pursue a career in the Army four years previously; my beloved and I were not as active in our social life as we should have been – a myriad reasons why. Friendships were slipping and life was passing by in an effortless blur. Busy

completing my certification requirements to become an ARTbundance™ Coach and Practitioner, I was looking forward to shaking up my business and my own staid, dull life.

"The day after I graduated as a certified ARTbundance™ Coach and Practitioner, I was getting dressed after showering. Applying body lotion to my breasts, I felt a definite lump on my left breast, toward the armpit.

"Hmmmmm. Hadn't I felt something a lot smaller two weeks ago, but then got busy with 'stuff'? Immediately I felt sick. Oh my goodness. My beloved maternal grandmother died of breast cancer when I was ten years old and as I lived with her, the whole 'cancer spectre' haunted me throughout my life. My fears of thirty years had come true. I had breast cancer. I rang my doctor's surgery (it was Friday) and they gave me an appointment to see my GP in ten days' time, which I duly accepted. I shared my discovery with my mum and my beloved, but not my fears.

"On the following Monday morning, I rang back the surgery and insisted I see a doctor immediately (given my family history of breast cancer). My GP tried to reassure me that it was probably a cyst – especially as I had undertaken two private DITI (Digital Infrared Thermal Imaging) tests in November 2010 and March 2011, which had been reported as clear, and had undergone a course of deep tissue massage on the back of those results. The GP's secretary managed to secure a cancellation appointment at the Breast Care Clinic for the following week. Thank you, angels!

"The breast care nurse specialist laid me down and took two syringes of liquid to try to drain the 'cyst.' I tried

hard not to cry as I saw the syringes swirl with fluid mixed with a stream of blood. I knew exactly what that meant.

"An ultrasound scan followed and I knew, as soon as the doctor was called in to take a look at the screen, they had discovered cancer. The look of sadness and compassion in this doctor's eyes as she gently took my hand was too much for me to bear. I burst into tears, utterly heartbroken, while the doctor took five core biopsies, which caused the skin surrounding the biopsies to necrotize. With a raging infection and fever, I was placed on high-dosage antibiotics and requested to stay close to the hospital 'just in case.'

"Five days later, I succumbed to my idea of hell and meekly underwent a series of mammograms, which were followed by a further ultrasound scan and a biopsy of tissue on my right breast, too. Again, I knew from the look on the radiographer's face that this was no large cyst in my left breast. I knew from the word 'go' that I had breast cancer and that the diagnosis, and subsequent treatment, was not just going to turn MY life upside-down, but those of my loved ones too.

"Later that day came the news that I had waited 30 fearful years to hear: at the age of 40, I was diagnosed with breast cancer. The Macmillan nurse delivered two powerful blows: (1) I was definitely going to lose my waist-length ringlets, and (2) I would be sterile by the time chemotherapy finished with me. Those were my words, not hers, by the way! She shared this life-changing news far more gently. I was also given a leaflet by the breast care nurse specialist, which detailed the support offered by a local breast cancer *charity, The Haven, which was to be a lifeline of support for me as I progressed through treatment.*

"Submitted for a volley of further exploratory tests over the next few days, plus emergency visits to a new dentist to get my mouth ready for chemo-aggravation, this was the longest week of my life. I was so afraid that my deep tissue massage treatment had spread the cancer cells throughout my lymph nodes and beyond...but thankfully test results showed that no, there was no metastasis. However, the tumour was not oestrogen-receptive as they had suspected, but Triple Negative (TNBC), which meant the whole shebang of treatment was needed and immediate surgery to remove the fast-growing aggressive tumour.

"I had no doubt I would get through the treatment and go on to live a very happy, healthy life, although the idea of going through intensive treatment terrified me. There was no room in my world for anything other than positive thinking, even during chemotherapy when my body reacted very strongly to interference! The overwhelming feeling that my life was meant to be lived as a joyfully loving experience, through laughter and play, saw me taking time out and restructuring my entire life – and my business – to support my new vision of life.

"My treatment began with a lumpectomy, followed by a follow-up appointment with my amazing onco-plastic surgeon who presented three options: mastectomy, re-excision (known as a 'scrape'), or leave it and undergo more radiotherapy treatments after chemotherapy. My answer was immediate: re-excision, please. The operation went well, as did the recovery from the surgery. Chemo wasn't so easy: the nausea, dental

pain, back pain, dangerously high blood pressure. My body was fighting cardiac toxicity, but with a slew of antibiotics, I felt very lucky to be alive after an all-too-close-brush with death.

"Yes, I lost my hair. On Day 17 of my first of four chemo cycles, it started to fall out. Although I was devastated at losing my hair, I had it cut short to a curly pixie-cut, which I loved. On Day 20 of chemo, our local hairdresser shaved off my hair. Surprisingly, I burst into fits of giggles when I saw myself – I looked just my dad! I felt so liberated!"

Callie is an inspiration, a muse. Her outlook on her situation was that it was nothing more than a blip on the movie screen of her life, certainly nothing that would interfere with the rest of her life. She had too much to do, too much laughter and playfulness in her heart to spread around. Her "bubbliness" was very contagious. I feel it when talking to her whether via email, Skype or any other means of communication we use (she lives in the UK and I in the States).

"Laughter and a very dry sense of humour also helped pull me through.... I also planned on my world domination...he he! No, seriously, I just kept focusing on all the playful, delightful things I wished to do when I was fully fit and able again...time to be loud, proud and very playful!"

A positive attitude brings optimism into your life, even in the direst situations. It makes it easier to avoid the worry and negative thinking. If you adopt it as a way of life, great things can come your way. We all have setbacks in our life. They challenge us to be better, stronger and wiser. A true test of your attitude toward the obstacle you've encountered, whether you understand why it happened or not, is to be thankful and then move forward. Feel empowered in your ability to see it as a gift for the soul to help you grow bigger than you ever thought you could. You'll have more energy, more happiness. You'll be able to surmount most any difficulty with grace. You'll develop a stronger sense of inner power. And like Callie, you will be able to inspire and motivate yourself and others. Life will smile at you.

"I look positively toward the next stage of my recovery – a complete and prophylactic bilateral mastectomy and immediate reconstruction in 2013. I have spent enough time in solitary reflection and completing in-depth research to accept and embrace wholeheartedly the changes that have happened in my miracle of a body that I am so blessed to be partnered with."

I believe gratitude and attitude go hand in hand. When we are grateful for our blessings and can maintain an optimistic attitude through thick and thin, there's no limit to the opportunities that will present themselves to us. When one door closes, a new one opens. Life IS meant to be good!

EXERCISE

We are going to make a Gratitude jar. Get a jar and mark it "Gratitude Jar." Every time something good happens in your life, write the date that it happened and a brief description on a piece of paper, and put it in the jar. Do it for a three-month period, or however long you wish to do it. Ideally, start the Gratitude jar at the beginning of the year and fill it for the whole year. When that period ends, open the jar and read about all the wonderful things that have happened during that time. Then celebrate all the good things in your life!

If you prefer to make it a Gratitude "box," get a shoebox and cut a 3 x 1/2 inch slit in the top of the box. Decorate the box as you wish and do the exercise above.

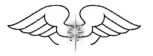

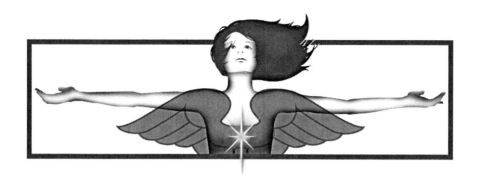

Establishing a Support System

> *"Support from family and friends, and communion with our own inner sacredness, are so important as we make our way through our healing.... It can be the difference between you feeling adrift and alone, and feeling empowered in your recovery."*

One week after my conversation with the therapist about how far I had come in my recovery (see "Gratitude and Attitude"), I participated in a 5K (3 1/2-mile) run – the Rudolph Fun Run – right before Christmas. Of course, I only walked! Now, understand that before I participated, I was only able to walk one mile before my leg gave way. So you can imagine how hard it was for me to go the full distance in the run. But go the full 5K, I did!

What kept me going after that first mile was the support I got from the owner of the rehab center I attended. She (and a friend of hers) walked with me every step of the way, encouraging me to keep going. When I thought I would collapse, they kept my attention on the goal of finishing. When I finally made it to the finish line, all the therapists who had participated in the run were there congratulating me on my victory. And what a victory it was for me! A huge milestone! I was one of only three patients with major traumas who had taken part in the run, and I had made it. It made me realize that we are the only ones who hold ourselves back from doing anything we want in our lives.

It's about letting go of those fears and resultant limiting beliefs we have that prevent us from taking steps forward in our lives (see "Limiting Beliefs"). I didn't think I would make it to the finish line, but I did, because of the support I had. Our personal journeys are our own and no one else can do it for us, but there's something to be said about having cheerleaders emboldening you to press ever onward.

A day after the run, I had another one of my epiphanies. I seemed to have a lot of those since my stroke. One other reason for my stroke being a gift from the gods was all the wisdom I gained.

I started thinking about my chapter on limiting beliefs. As I fell into the great waters of the feminine, going to the place within where the Great Mother, the archetype of the inner feminine essence, resides and where self-love is born, I realized I was still fearful of full recovery. What came to me again was that if I fully recovered, I wouldn't be taken care of as I had been for the time that my mom supported and cared for me.

Mom worked full-time as a university professor, teaching classes and grading all the students' assignments and tests, in addition to writing papers for publication. She was busy indeed, with school and domestic responsibilities; and then she had to care for *me*. But she took care of my every need, which in the beginning was everything from feeding me to bathing me, taking me to all my appointments, etc. As I became more self-sufficient, her care-giving duties became less and less, until the time where I was helping her.

We all want to be nurtured and cared for, and I've always needed that, even though I considered myself to be independent and strong. What I realized is that although I was being supported and cared for by someone outside myself, it was equally important to be cared for by my own inner femininity, that part of everyone that is the nurturing Great Mother, the inner maternal archetype. I feel that the work I was doing before my stroke – my healing arts business, working primarily with women – was the initial step of my transition, the first stepping stone of my journey to wholeness, where the masculine and feminine work in harmony to create inner balance. Now, almost two years and one stroke later, I had visited that inner sanctum where I sat on Great Mother's lap, embraced by her unconditional love, and I knew I had come home.

Support from family and friends, and communion with our own inner sacredness, are so important as we make our way through our healing. Sandi's story below shows just how much of an impact support can have on a person's recovery.

"My trauma began with the death of my mother at the age of 12, followed by several other childhood traumas. I was a depressed teenager, and I began to drink alcoholically [almost immediately]. I was an alcoholic before my very first episode of drinking. What I mean is that I had the mentality of a drinker from my earliest years and I never knew what would happen after I took that first drink.

"My drinking escalated until, by the time I was 38, I was drinking a quart of vodka a day. By this time I had a baby girl to take care of, and I wanted to stop, but I couldn't. I was physically, emotionally and spiritually addicted to alcohol. It was my god. I've been told that Carl Jung, the great psychologist from the 20th century, said that alcoholics are spiritual people searching for their spirituality, using the wrong spirits. This describes my affliction precisely: I was drinking my life away, looking for the answers in the bottom of a bottle, knowing I couldn't find them there.

63

"I finally found my way to a particular recovery meeting that I could stand after almost having lost my baby to Child Protective Services. I was contemptuous of recovery, as many people are, prior to investigation. But there was nowhere else to go. It was there that I learned to manage to live, not just one day at a time, but one moment at a time. Once I detoxed myself (and detoxing is a hideous experience), I could push back the urge for a drink one moment at a time. There were many lessons that I learned, and continue to learn, from recovery. The one thing that comes to mind is that alcoholics all drink to change the way they feel. It comes down to that. We are a group of people who normally would not mix, but are bound together by this devastating, uniquely physical, emotional, and spiritual disease. Through the support of the recovery meetings, I have found a way to live in humility and integrity.

"What got me through the ordeal of learning to live a sober life were the people in the rooms of the recovery meetings, loving me unconditionally until, and even after, I learned to love myself.

"My life has had its dreary moments. Just because I gave up drinking doesn't mean my addictive personality went away. There are many other ways to 'stuff' your feelings – eating, shopping, relationships, sex – any number of things. I was an eater, shopper, and 'stuck' in a very unhealthy relationship. The eating developed into a severe case of bulimia, the shopping led me into financial debt and the dead relationship in which I was immersed with another alcoholic living in his disease...they were all ways of filling up the god-sized hole in my heart.

"Through therapy and recovery, I have found the courage to begin letting go of all the material things of this world – by this, I mean anything that is not of the spirit.... Recovery offers a life you never thought possible – a life of spirit and spirituality without using the wrong spirits."

I have an interesting tale to relate about another perspective on support. As I was listening to a webinar on starting to market essential oils (another interest of mine), my mind started wandering (so what's new!). As the speakers in the webinar were giving their spiel, I was thinking, "Why do I want to listen to this? I already know what they're trying to teach me." I had been involved in network marketing endeavors before, but unsuccessfully. So why was I doing it again? Then another thought crossed my mind. It was one of envy and judgment. The speakers were very successful in their business; they were where I wanted to be in my endeavors, but I hadn't gotten there yet. I was still burdened by the fears that held me back from taking off.

As I dug deeper into my feelings, I had another revelation. I thought of all the people I had been meeting online through social networking. So many were touting their wares, putting themselves out on the market, gaining a strong following and establishing themselves as experts in their respective fields. I envied them and found myself judging them because I saw them as "arrogant," claiming to be more enlightened than they really were. Where the heck was that coming from? I kept digging and what came to me was this: these people were actually a huge part of my support system. Now, you're probably wondering, "What the heck is she saying? Part of her support group?" Support comes from people encouraging you, loving you, standing by you in your time of need. How did these people fit into my support structure?

It was like this. They were a trigger for feelings I never thought I had, so in an "indirect" way, they were supporting me by helping me bring old hidden thoughts and beliefs to the surface, where I could work through them and release them into the ether so they were no longer part of my life. Thus, I was moving further forward along the path to full recovery. I have to say, as I've said before, this book was instrumental in my healing. With each chapter I wrote, the theme was what I needed to work on at that moment. I guess I had to understand that support isn't just from those who surround you with love and compassion. It also comes indirectly from those who bring out the worst in you so you can clear yourself of the negativity that keeps you from fulfilling your purpose on Earth. Maybe I will find the abundance I dream of, after all!

Creating and maintaining a support system is important during your recovery. Your loved ones and all the other supportive people in your life provide the love, warmth and connection you need. Sometimes, those relationships are a primary source of motivation. When I walked in the 5K run, it was the therapists' encouragement that kept me going, just as the people at the recovery organization kept Sandi moving forward through her recovery. While you are responsible for your own recovery, part of being responsible is knowing when and who to ask for help. And that means also turning inward and asking for Divine guidance. A strong support system can be the difference between you feeling adrift and alone, and feeling empowered in your recovery.

"I have a chance for a new life. I'm living with a lot of pain and depression right now, even after 13 years of sobriety. I am feeling feelings I thought were long dead, and even ones I never knew I had. The disease has long tentacles. It affects everything. However, I am now a viable member of society, well-educated, a school teacher, and home-owner. I have a fairly well-adjusted daughter whom I hope to send to college in a year.

"Money is a big problem, but when I look back on my life as a drunken woman living in poverty, I know I've been re-born and given another chance at life.... I have work that is hard but rewarding – I'm considered an excellent teacher in a 'good' school. I own my own home, old and ramshackle as it may be, which I share with five sweet pets and a beloved daughter. I think part of that daughter's mission in this life was to save me. We have survived our lives fairly intact to this point. I hope and expect we will always have a loving relationship. I write and teach writing to children during summers. It's not a bad life, but I do struggle, and my hope is that it will get easier."

Don't try to go through your recovery alone. We don't live in a vacuum in the world. We are all connected in this great big Universe and are meant to help our fellow (wo)man. Reach out for help whenever and wherever you need it. There will always be someone there to help you in your time of need. Surround yourself with loving people who will be there for you, but don't forget to go within to seek solace, too, from the sacred maternal nurturer inside yourself. And always look at how other people may be a reflection of you, compelling you to purge any negative energy that may be preventing you from being all you are meant to be. "In our connection is our strength. The bonds that connect us are ones of loving spirituality...what we do affects one another.... A person can survive the worst and heal if they are aware of loving and being loved."[17]

EXERCISE

In your journal or notebook, write down all those people who make up your support system and the ways they support you. Include those who trigger negativity in you and what it is that they are triggering in you. If you need support, find out if there is a local support group in your area that can help. Check local hospitals and online resources.

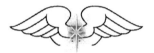

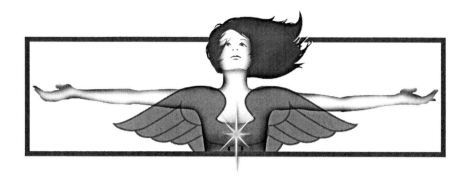

Surrendering:
Letting Go and Letting God

"When we surrender to God – the omnipotent, omniscient, and omnipresent power in all of us – magic happens."

S urrender...let go! I hear that all the time.

In books: "Surrender is the simple but profound wisdom of yielding to rather than opposing the flow of life...to surrender is to accept the present moment unconditionally and without reservation."[18]

On social networking sites: "Surrendering to possibility is an admission that we do not know everything and cannot see the future. It is also an invitation for newer, higher, yet unknown solutions, opportunities and synchronicities to emerge."[19]

On blogs: "We are all, in our own way, afloat on the...river of life. To surrender doesn't mean to throw out the paddles. It does mean to work with the flow to get to our destination. When we surrender, we can easily prioritize and act in ways that use the flow, rather than fight against it. We can use our paddles to push off the rocks when the timing is right, rather than paddle furiously upstream only to get blindsided by the rock when we inevitably hit it because we didn't act wisely with the flow."[20]

In newspapers: "Surrender is what we look forward to when we notice we are holding on, or what we look back on and assess when we realize what we let go of, maybe when inquiring deeper, what dropped away. But when we are here, we are there. Where is the 'other' to go? There is nowhere that 'Source' isn't."[21]

At the end of 2012, as we were entering a new era of consciousness, it only stood to reason that this was the best time to surrender, letting go of the past. And as always, as I continued my recovery, the message came when I was really ready to listen. I had already been led by my psyche to heed other messages, which I then explored in the previous chapters of this book and would continue to do so until I had heard all the messages I was to hear, presenting them in future chapters. I was now ready to take on the task of "surrendering and letting go." But first I had to know what that meant to me. The image that appeared as I dwelled on this was me floating down the Guadalupe River in the Texas Hill Country on a tube. Now, if you know anything about tubing down a river, it's very peaceful as you quietly glide along the water, sailing without a rudder, until you encounter the tumultuous rapids where you dip and dive and are tossed around. You have to be very careful lest you run up against the craggy rocks jutting up from the river bed, or you are submerged in the depths by the strong tide.

I wasn't sure at first why this image came up when thinking of surrender, because to be caught in the rapids requires much focus and physical and mental maneuvering to be able to pass through the turbulence and move back to the serenity of the quietly flowing water.

But that was it! That's what surrendering meant to me. It meant that when I was navigating a stormy time in my life, I needed to do my share of the work getting through – with focused attention and appropriate actions – and then let go and surrender to the Universe, which would help carry me through the rough period and guide me to the ensuing peaceful waters. Remember we are co-creators with the Higher Powers. As we do our part in our lives to grow into our personal power – usually through the trials and tribulations of turbulent times – Spirit is always there giving us all the support we need to carry through and carry on.

When I talk about Spirit or the Universe or our co-creator, I speak of the God-like essence that is within each of us. It's our own divinity that connects us to each other, to all of nature. Remember my mantra "I am on a magic carpet ride with Spirit at the helm"? Life's journey is full of magic – the marvelous, the miraculous and the wonderful – but it's not without its hurdles along the way. And when we come to these bumps in the road, we need to have faith and believe that the Universe "has our back" and will be our pillar of strength, propping us up and propelling us forward.

Kim's story below illustrates that strong faith in the power of God and the Universe, and what it brings forth in one's life when one listens to the Divine messages.

"At the beginning of the year I had many doubts, insecurities and lack of belief in anything I had in my life. I felt for some reason like a stranger and I had become the very thing that would seem to crush my artistic abilities. I had become a normal run-of-the-mill everybody kind of person. Not that there's anything wrong with that, but for me it felt like all my dreams, desires and ambitions had been depleted and before I knew what was happening, massive depression set in.

"Doing projects that have creative and artistic meaning sets the mood for me. I have learned over recent years that all artists suffer from a lack of creativity. The problem wasn't that I lacked the ability but that I wasn't taking care of my mental, physical and spiritual self,

which squelched the desire and any creativity from flowing.

"So I began to feel worthless and unwanted, especially when someone to whom I confided my feelings betrayed me. This person acted as if none of what I said mattered and before it was all over, I was broken. By February, I knew something had to change or I was going to die.

"I come from an amazing church, The Seed Church in Savannah, Georgia, and we are a strong faith-and-move-of-God type of church. To top it all off, I'm a praise leader and have a strong presence in every aspect of our church. In the nearly 20 years I have been there, I have never been so broken – and yet I wanted to die.

"The problem was that I have two amazing children, Ceron, 11 and Kegan, 6. How could I leave these two? But the thought of being over this pain, that the tears of insanity I faced every day would all be gone and I would be in heaven, was a welcome thought since peace would finally take over what was so missing inside of me.

"So one stormy February day, I sat in my house with not a soul around. My husband, Sean, was at work and my kids were at school. I took one of our handguns, loaded it and headed outside to our shed to do the deed. My cell phone dinged with a text from the very person who betrayed me. This person was broken and so sorry for what had happened and it melted my heart.

"For some crazy reason, I told her what was going on and she called and spent the day on the phone with me, making sure I was okay. My friend convinced me to call my husband to tell him. He rushed home from work to make sure I didn't pull the trigger and made me call my

pastor to have her pray for me. Pastor Datha not only prayed but had me come to prayer group that night. It was the moment I was set free.

"I still struggled with the loss and hopelessness that I felt, and the lack of connectedness I had with the people in my life. I knew all of this was me, but why? As time went on, I had to stop everything I was doing and fight. I had to fight for my life and had to maintain a will to stay alive. I then stopped all activities in my business and even in church. I spent time with God and surrounded myself with people who loved and prayed with me.

"It was fight or die! For me, there were no in-betweens. I knew what I had to do: I had to spend time on me. I learned the source of my crash was years of taking care of everything and everyone else. Not being myself, the time came when all I had to give was no more. I realized that if I was going to succeed in all God had [planned] for me, the most important thing was staying connected to Him and taking care of myself."

For Kim, surrendering meant letting go of the notion that she had to be all things to all people, and by taking care of herself, she could fulfill her life's purpose as directed by God.

"Through the power of prayer and being connected to God...I feel better and more alive now than I did as a result of doing it God's way. Making sure I was taking care of myself and being more selfish in a good way helped me get past this. I learned that before you can do anything for family or anyone else, you have to take care of yourself."

Eckhart Tolle says the following about surrender (or non-surrender, as the case may be) in his book *The Power of Now:* "Non-surrender hardens your psychological form, the shell of

73

the ego, and so creates a strong sense of separateness.... Not only your psychological form but also your physical form – your body – becomes hard and rigid through resistance."[22]

How uncanny that I opened to that page as I was writing this chapter. For the last week of December 2012, my body had become very stiff and unwieldy, or should I say, my right stroked side had. I could barely walk or use my right arm. My hand and fingers felt like they didn't belong to me, and I felt like a zombie from the heaviness of the stroke. It was as if I wasn't of this planet. I moved about ever so slowly, trying to make my right leg move like a normal limb, and my arm just dangled by my side with very little strength to do much of anything. Was all the rehab and exercise I had done for naught? Geez, only a few weeks before, I had walked three-and-a-half miles in the Rudolf Fun Run! So what was going on?

As I was still lying in bed on New Year's Eve morning at 10:00 am (which was unheard of for me considering I used to get up when the rooster crowed every morning), I thought of something. Another illumination revealing itself? While I lay there, cozy and warm under the covers, my body luxuriating in nothingness, my mind chattered away. My monkey mind flitted from one thought to another, thinking about all I had to do when the New Year began: updating my website and my blog, setting up my crowd-funding campaign for this book, finishing the book, getting back to my sacred feminine community and my Yin Radiance program that I had abandoned, launching my book, and getting a house and car, among other things. Was I going to be able to do it all? I mean, I wasn't even fully recovered yet and I didn't know when I would be.

My energy level was very low and I was still operating at a snail's pace. It was this old, frenetic mindset that was causing my body and mind to be rigid. Once again, I was resisting the natural flow of life by trying to control things in my mind and worrying because I didn't know how I would physically be able to achieve what I needed to do. I was in bondage by my thoughts. I guess I hadn't quite gotten rid of the masculine-driven, ego- and fear-based mentality that had contributed to my stroke. It's not easy to purge those negative characteristics and behaviors that have plagued one for years, or centuries if you believe we've lived many lives before. And my body was feeling the impact of my resistance to letting go of this mindset.

I needed to surrender where I could "see clearly what needs to be done...[taking action]...doing one thing at a time and focusing on one thing at a time."[23] I didn't need to force things to happen or worry about when things would get done. Everything has its own Divine timing. I needed to surrender and reconnect with the source-energy of just Being, the co-creator of my life, the creator of all life. If we watch the magnificence that is created by the Divine, we can learn from the natural flow of life. We see how the miracles of life unfold naturally without fear, without manipulation, without force or resistance.

When we surrender to God, the omnipotent, omniscient and omnipresent power in all of us, magic happens. We are no longer dictated by external conditions, but by our own inner grace and spirit. We no longer react or resist or act from a conditioned monkey mind. When we are in the presence of this inner personal power, we are transformed, and when we are transformed, our world is transformed, because the world is only a reflection, a macrocosm of our microcosm. Just think if all people would surrender to the power of the Universe. There would be no separateness, only connectedness to the source of all creation and to each other. It would be heaven on earth!

EXERCISE:

In your journal or notebook, write down ways you can surrender to the Higher Powers that will make your circumstances easier to get through. What thoughts or behaviors can you turn over to this Higher Power? When things get difficult, "Let go and let God."

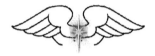

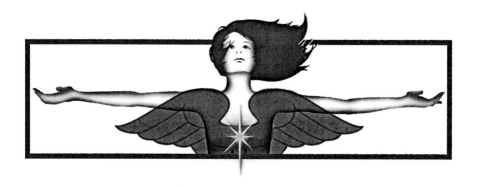

Believing in Yourself

> *"Believing in yourself doesn't come from others or outer circumstances. It comes from within. It's about having self-love.... It's about knowing that no matter what your situation, you have the wherewithal to meet that challenge head on and deal with it."*

I've already briefly discussed the subject of "believing in yourself" in the context of "never giving up," but I wish to talk more fully about it here, beginning with another story of my progress at the rehab center. It was the first week in January 2013 and my first physical therapy session of the year. My therapist was a wonderful young man (young enough to be my son) who not only was a fantastic therapist with tremendous wisdom, but he had a beautiful loving soul as well. I would say he had a great inner balance between the masculine and feminine principles. He knew when to be firm and demanding, and when to be compassionate and nurturing.

Since this session was the first of the year and I hadn't been for a month, it was time to do an evaluation of where I was in my recovery so he could determine what kind of program to create for the next stretch of my recovery. We discussed where I was in my recovery; he made a point to mention my success in the 5K Fun Run. He then asked me what I wanted as my goals. Of course, my overall goal was "full recovery," but on an emotional level, I wanted to return to something that was near and dear to me: salsa dance lessons.

Having been a ballet dancer for ten years in my younger years, dancing was part of my soul. Over my last couple of months in rehab in 2012, my therapist had me doing some very basic salsa dance steps as part of my exercise. In fact, the music they played at the rehab center was often salsa music, which made my hips twitch whenever it was on. Then he told me *his* goals for me. Oh my gosh! They were some lofty goals.

"Erica, I want you to build up to thirty minutes on the elliptical." Never mind that I had never done more than ten minutes on that godforsaken machine, even before my stroke. Then he proceeded to tell me all the exercises we were going to work on over the next few months. I think he wanted to turn me into Superwoman by the end!

Sitting on the mat, peering at him with a subdued sense of amazement (I didn't want him to think I wasn't willing to work that hard!), I just agreed with his plan, but in my monkey mind, all I could hear was, "How the heck am I going to be able to withstand being on the elliptical for thirty minutes?"

Unfortunately, my therapist could read right through me. He could tell that behind my calm countenance lay dread. And then he said it, those simple words that turned my world around at that moment – "Believe in yourself, Erica! You can do it. Look at what you accomplished in the 5K Fun Run. Before, you couldn't walk but a mile, but you did 3 1/2 miles that day."

It was true. I could barely walk one mile when I did my regular walk around the neighborhood. But with the support of the therapy team cheering me on at the Fun Run, I reached a huge milestone in my recovery (of course, I went into a physical coma for a week afterward!). And it was time again to reach another.

"I don't care if you could only go ten minutes before on the elliptical," my therapist stated firmly. "That was the past. This is NOW! And this is what I want you to work toward." He was asserting his authority as my healer; he knew what I could do and he was going to push me, to make me go beyond my limits. "You probably won't like me; you may even hate me." But I could never hate him. I knew he was doing it for my own good. I wanted to recover fully. He wanted the same. But there was a difference between us. He believed in me more than I believed in myself. Although I had a strong determination and perseverance, I also succumbed to my weakness, to the notion that I was physically delicate like my father had been (he passed away at 50 years old).

But wasn't 2013 the beginning of the era of transformation? Wasn't my stroke the means through which I was to morph into a whole new person? Those three words – "believe in yourself" – stuck with me for weeks to come. I went to bed at night reciting them as my mantra. I created a picture with the words "Believe in Yourself and Watch the Miracle Unfold" and posted it on my Facebook fan page. And I wrote this chapter! It was time for me to start believing in myself – REALLY believing in all I could do and all I could offer. My deepest gratitude goes to my therapist for helping me see the greatness in me that would continue to propel me toward my full recovery.

Believing in yourself doesn't come from others or outer circumstances. It comes from within. It's about having self-love. It's about knowing you have something to offer the world – your special gift, whatever it may be. It's about knowing that no matter what your situation, you have the wherewithal to meet that challenge head on and deal with it.

No one can devalue you; only you can do that to yourself. If you can hold your head high no matter what someone says to or about you, or what the circumstances are, you can quiet those inner gremlins that try to sabotage you by making you feel unworthy. Elisabeth Kübler Ross said, "People are like stained glass windows. They sparkle and shine when the sun is out, but when the darkness sets in, their true beauty is revealed only if there is light within."

As I said before, you are not your life situation. You can make your life what you want it to be by believing in yourself. You become what you want to become based on what your inner guidance speaks to you about your desires and passions.

Read how Cindy overcame the limitations of Multiple Sclerosis by believing in herself, by not having the victim's "Oh, woe is me!" attitude, and by having the mindset that her condition doesn't make her who she is.

"'Don't tell anyone I said this, but you have multiple sclerosis.' The words flew out of his mouth as lethal as bullets. The elderly ophthalmologist was disgruntled because I had made an appointment to see him without first seeing an optometrist and this would likely send his billing into chaos.

"I sat there with my pupils dilated from the eye drops he'd administered, shocked and scared. 'Multiple sclerosis?' My 28-year-old brain raced to make sense of this. All I could come up with was Jerry Lee Lewis and the children in wheelchairs. I knew this was not good.

"As I was driving home that rainy, grey fall day, the tears poured down my face as fast as the wipers washed away the rain. The lights of the oncoming cars blurred into orbs, my heartbeat pulsed in my ears. With every rainy mile, my hopes and dreams for the future fell away. I was having an out-of-body experience – so much so that I failed to see the car that I almost hit until it blared its horn at me.

"In that single moment in the doctor's chair, I had become one ugly word. I had become a 'patient.' I had become a victim. I had become a burden to my loved ones. I would no longer be the woman I knew myself to be.

"I somehow managed to make the 20-minute drive on that rainy afternoon out of the city to my suburban bungalow. My husband was still at work and my eight-year-old son was still in school. I was alone. Alone and scared as I sat on the kitchen floor and cried. Cried tears of fear, tears for the loss of my dreams and tears for my son who would now have to deal with having a sick mother.

"As human nature dictates, I did the most natural thing in the world. I called my mother, who then lived three hours away. I wanted my mom to make everything alright again. But she could not help. No one could.

"I remember when I was a little girl and my mother would hold my hands and dance with me in the living room. I thought she was beautiful with her lip-sticked red lips and shiny auburn hair. She would always sing her favorite song, 'Que sera, sera, whatever will be, will be.' Whenever I heard her hum this, it filled me with dreams of what wonderful things lay ahead. Somehow this was not what I had envisioned when I was a girl of five. This was not the happily ever after I thought my mother was singing about.

"My vision started to blur when I was 28. I was a young mother married to a traveling businessman and working as a clerk in the accounting department of a law firm. I first noticed my blurry vision on a weekend getaway with my husband to a friend's wedding. We had planned this trip for months, looking forward to having

81

some alone time away from the responsibilities of work and parenting. The wedding was in another city, a six-hour drive away. On that Friday night drive, as the sun began to set over a farmer's field of wheat, I noticed my vision in my right eye was smudged, as if someone had rubbed a pat of butter across my eyeball. The beautiful sunset that normally would have soothed me instead filled me with an eerie sense of foreboding, which was with me the entire weekend. It was a third partner on the dance floor, an invisible presence in our hotel bed. I could not shake the sense that something unwanted was stalking me.

"*After returning home, my vision returned to normal and life as I knew it resumed. Until it happened again, and this time I could not pretend it was nothing to worry about. Work became difficult. Working with numbers all day in accounting strained the bad eye. This led me to the elderly, insensitive ophthalmologist who spat out my diagnosis without any compassion for my situation – a young woman with a future ahead of me and my child to worry about.*

"*I had my first son at the early age of 20 and I suffered a miscarriage when I was 24, which devastated me. I wanted to have another child before it was too late, but I knew having a baby with multiple sclerosis was a risky venture. But I took the gamble and became pregnant. I was thrilled. I reveled in my growing belly and never felt better than during my pregnancy. MS was, in the meantime, a distant monster.*

"*After 12 hours [of labor], my beautiful son was born. He looked like an angel. Sweet, innocent, and perfect. I felt like he was a gift from God and I felt blessed each time I looked into his sky blue eyes. I thanked God each time I held him, as I stood in front of the sun-filled window and looked out at the beautiful fall leaves. I thought should I die [in that instant], I had been blessed with this second miracle.*

"But my fairy tale moment of bliss came to a crashing end. Just days after my new baby's arrival, my vision in my one eye not only blurred but blacked to nothingness. I was blind in one eye. My husband did not believe me until he shined a flashlight into my eye and I didn't even flinch. I was scared, lost in my own darkness. I made a deal with God that day as I lay on my bed with my two-week-old son. I was terrified at the thought of not being able to see him grow up. What would he look like at one, three, or as a man? I bargained with God, 'Please let me see just long enough for me to see what he looks like when he is five.' It was the darkest time of my life – literally and emotionally.

"Over the next few years, my self-image was shattered from the many doses of steroids to treat my MS that inevitably led to an extra 20 pounds of weight. I had always defined myself in terms of my sex appeal. In my teenage years, I was hot and I knew it. On my wedding day, I was a tiny 98 pounds. And I now found myself at an unrecognizable weight. Who was that in the mirror? Surely it could not be me, my inner voice would cry out. When my ex-husband bought me a pair of running shoes and a yoga mat for my birthday two weeks before he said he wanted a divorce, my self-confidence hit rock bottom.

"This caused me to look within and find who I really was. It was not the makeup or hair that made me lovable. It was not the skinny jeans that validated me. Being confident in who you are, willing to love with an

open heart, and accepting life as it comes are not things you can find in the makeup aisle.

"I have merged my teenage self with my unrecognizable self and now love what I see in the mirror: a happy, confident, secure woman who knows who she is and loves herself unconditionally.

"My vision today has still not fully recovered, but I am thankful for what vision I have and do not dwell on what I don't have. I am happy to say my second-born is now 17 and a handsome young man who still has beautiful sky blue eyes that I can 'see.' I just recently held my first grandson, who peered up at me with his blue eyes, and I smiled. Smiled at the beauty that is life. Smiled at the gifts we are given each day if we are only willing to see them. We judge what we think we 'see,' not what is the deeper truth.

"I am now happy with who I am and love the Cindy that is ever-evolving. My vision may be flawed, but I see more clearly now than I ever have.

"Multiple sclerosis is not who I am. It is what I have. MS does not define me, but is a small part of what makes up who I am. My spirit has not diminished, but shines as brightly as the northern star. Look up and see the shining 'me.'

"I know that whatever the future brings, I will be okay. That I am strong enough in spirit to accept what is. I believe that every day we are given is a gift. I believe we all have the ability not only to overcome obstacles, but to grow even richer in our understanding of our true self.

"I might still fall flat on my face, but I will always get right back up and brush off the dirt. I might not laugh if

it hurts, but I will still smile at my ability to not feel defeated, knowing that next time, I just might see that curb in the nick of time. If I see you on the street, just call out my name and I will wave. I will see you. But will you see 'me'?

"You were right all along, Mom: 'whatever will be, will be.'"

To believe in yourself, you must first know yourself. Find your true essence, who you are at the center of your being. When you can transcend your self-doubts and fears that cloud your perception of who you truly are, you have reached that place of self-love. It is here that you realize your outer circumstance is not who you are; it is but a shadow that has darkened your path. And by shining a light on it, by embracing it as an ally and not an adversary, you empower yourself to detach from any misgivings that it may incite in you. In this state of great prowess, you begin to believe in the fabulous unique person that you are, and that you have a true purpose on Earth. Believe in yourself and "watch the miracle unfold."

EXERCISE

Get out your journal or notebook and write down all your positive attributes in the form of "I am _____" or "I have _____" or "I can (do) _____" or whatever way you can affirm the greatness you have inside. Then whenever you start questioning your worth, repeat whichever attributes are called for at that moment.

~ OR ~

Come up with your own mantra about believing in yourself. Make a poster of it, or make several and put them in every room where you live. Repeat them at night before going to sleep, and in the morning just before you get out bed. Repeat them whenever you think about them throughout the day.

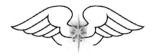

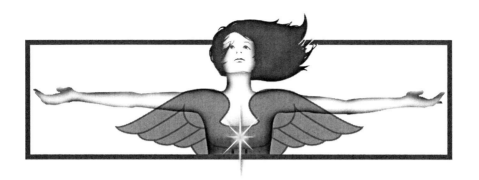

Living in the Moment

> *"If you're living in the present, you're living in acceptance of what is, realizing that everything is complete as it is. By living in the present, you have the power to change your life."*

I seemed to have fallen into a routine when I went to sleep at night. I would go to bed around 10 or 11 pm because I was usually exhausted by then, and I would fall asleep fairly easily. I would wake up about two hours later because nature called (sorry for "too much information"!). Since I use my phone as my alarm, it would be next to me in my bed, which I know is not a good thing since it emits radiation that messes with our sleep cycles. Nonetheless, it would lie there with me in its own "snooze" mode, since I would mute its sound so, other than the alarm, it wouldn't wake me up when emails came through or I received messages from someone on Facebook or a text message or whatever.

The problem was that if I was awakened by nature, which usually happened more than once (sorry for TMI again!), I would check my phone once I crawled back into bed to see if I had received any sort of messages, and I'd even respond if I felt compelled to (I know that's crazy, but that's the way I am). And then, of course, I would be wide awake and my monkey mind would start chattering away, thinking of all I had to do for my crowd-funding project and my book launch, and then I would start to panic over whether I would be able to get it all done. Oh, woe is me! Wasn't night time when I was supposed to be getting my rest, so I could wake up refreshed in the morning for another day? But no, the mind chatter would continue, thinking about this and thinking about that. How could I shut it off? Of course, the more I tried with all my might to turn off my mind, the worse it would get. It's true that the thing you fear most will come upon you and overtake you.

Then I would think about Eckhart Tolle's book *The Power of Now*, and how one finds inner peace when living in the present moment – not in the past, not in the future, but in the "now." "As long as you are in a state of intense presence, you are free of thought."[24] So to help quiet my mind, I would lie on my side, putting my hands on either side of my head, and administer Reiki to myself. If you don't know what Reiki is, it's a Japanese technique of stress reduction and relaxation that also promotes healing. It is administered by "laying on hands," allowing the "life force energy" to pass through to where the energy is needed to revitalize and heal. I've been a Reiki master for about seven years now and love the benefits of the energy work. Each night I put my hands on my heart (my heart chakra) and my stomach (my solar plexus chakra) before falling asleep, to give myself a brief Reiki treatment. I used to have anxieties, as I talked about previously, which would make my heart flutter; and my stomach is where most of my anxieties would settle, causing digestive disturbances (TMI, I know!). Regularly giving myself Reiki, focusing on those two points, helped keep the anxieties at bay.

Well, as I was giving my head Reiki, which subdued the mental chatter, I was able to keep my mind free of thought and take myself out of my chaotic mental voyage, into the future and back to the present land of slumber, back to my dark bedroom, cozy under the covers. I would be transported back into the dream world of the night where I belonged. I was at peace and knew that all was as it should be, that I didn't have to worry about all that needed to be done. I was guided by Spirit, knowing I would not be led astray, that things would take their course without me having to worry about them.

We live in an age of distraction. We let the present slip away as we ruminate on our past or worry about the future. The world in which we live creates "mental fragmentation, disintegration, distraction and decoherence," as Buddhist scholar B. Alan Wallace puts it.

But life unfolds in the present. When you become more mindful of the present, you become an observer of your thoughts instead of "being" your thoughts. By just being with your thoughts, neither grasping at them nor pushing them away, you awaken to life's possibilities. No longer do you let your thoughts control you. No longer are you letting your life go by without living it each and every moment.

Get away from the "egoic mode of consciousness: identified with [your] mind and run by [your] mind"[25] As long as the egoic mind (or monkey mind, as I call it) runs your life, you cannot be truly at ease or at peace or fulfilled, since the ego identifies with external things and needs to be fed constantly.

When you seek yourself in the mind and mistake it for who you are, (e.g. when you're lost in thoughts about your life situation), you allow the egoic mind to create your reality. But it's a false reality based on fear: a fear that maybe your circumstances will never get better, a fear grounded in the future. The egoic mind cannot survive without strife and conflict. What you need to do to get out of this egoic state of consciousness is to reclaim consciousness from your mind and direct it to your "inner body," which connects you to the source of all creation. It is your true essence. By focusing your attention away from thinking and directing it onto your inner body, you move into a state of Being, where you are living in the present moment, in the "Now."

When I would find myself struggling with falling back to sleep at night, I would feel my inner body radiating from my head to my toes, drinking in the life force energy of Reiki, and I would peacefully drift off back to sleep.

Read now how Vanessa overcame her crippling anxieties by moving away from her thoughts and into her body, into the state of Being.

"I was having what I thought was a normal day, although it was a bit hectic because I was running the family from here to there. It was also my husband's birthday and I was trying to please him. I was feeling a bit overwhelmed, but I put on the happy face for all concerned. My husband popped in for a quick haircut, so I waited in the car with my three children out in the front. They were restless and I was unable to calm them. I then had a strange feeling in the back of my head and began to feel a bit nauseated. By the time my husband returned to the car, I felt terrible, with pins and needles in both my arms. I was beginning to be frightened, and my self-diagnosis was a stroke of some sort. My husband drove me to the local hospital and they saw me fairly quickly, and soon made their own diagnosis of a panic attack. By this time, I also had pins and needles up my legs and in my chest area.

"Now to some, this probably doesn't sound like a trauma, and I understand that people go through some amazing challenges. However, I am a very positive person and I have done a lot of personal growth work and work to understand the core of me. I am an intuitive and spiritual life coach, so how could I be having a panic attack? I couldn't believe I was so stressed that I could be having a panic attack. I dreamt up all sorts of other diseases I must have, which made me panic even more. My mind was taking control of everything I was doing

and over-exaggerating it all. I seemed unable to get myself out of the feeling that I was out of control. It was extremely daunting and concerning, and at one stage, I felt I was going to hide under the chair in the waiting room...totally irrational behavior.

"The doctor prescribed some medication, which seemed to take ages to work. All the time, I felt distant and isolated from the world. Although I was in the same room as the others, it just seemed I was locked inside my head, totally disconnected from them. I went home that night, aware that under-breathing or over-breathing could set off this reaction within me and would result in the pins and needles in my body.

"The next morning, trying to get out the door for the day, I had another attack, although I had totally different symptoms. It was as if various colours in the room were exaggerated and jumped out at me, affecting my eyes. My temperature changed and my skin oscillated between feeling burning hot and freezing cold. The feeling ran from the back of my neck right down my body and into my toes, a moment of temperature difference that was significantly palpable. I was once again frightened and told my husband I needed to go to the hospital again, as I felt so strange inside my head, which was kind of pounding with loud sounds. To understand this feeling, it was like turning up the intensity of every sensation and feeling I would normally have by 1,000. I felt very out of control. At the hospital once again, I was told that it was anxiety, another panic attack.

"And so I spent the following three to four months having more than one attack per day, some days, and also during the night. I remember a visit I made to a large *hardware warehouse. As I moved my way into the shop, the aisles seemed to extend and grow and there was just so much to look at. All the items on the shelves seemed to enter my head, and once again the colours affected my eyes, the temperature sensations ran through my body, and my breathing became shallow and fast.*

"During those interestingly challenging and frightening months, I refused to drive and I didn't even like showering with the door shut. When I went to my local doctor to seek some support and counseling, he asked me to explain how I was feeling, and I told him to look at my handbag. Inside was a total jumble of everything mixed and matched: coins were out of purses, there was rubbish, and nothing was in any order. I told him that was not me. I usually had everything in its place. I could tell I was out of control. I realized I really had to learn about flow and Being.

"The panic came when I thought about the future or recalled the past, or entered or participated in overwhelming situations and places with lots of people and lots of colours...too much for my mind to process. If I centered myself in the moment, with meditation or breathing, I was able to quell the sensations within my body. I also understood the full impact of fear, although I wasn't really sure what I was fearful of.

"I really learnt about the potential of me, both the positive potential and the negative potential...of how my thoughts had created my reality. I really learnt about balance and honouring myself and my knowing in every moment. My affirmation 'I'm in the right place at the right time, and I am safe' became my mantra for months on end. It really helped me to centre daily, hourly and

even in the minute, and find myself and love myself just there.

"I was on medication for a period of twelve months and slowly but surely, by practicing yoga and maintaining my presence in the moment, I noticed that the attacks I had been having became less intense and less frequent until I stopped having them for almost four months, at which time I finished the medication.

"I had been off the medication for about four months when one morning, once again a very busy morning in the house with lots happening – visitors staying and children needing things everywhere – I woke up feeling wrong. When my husband came home, I told him I wanted to go back to the doctor before things got out of hand, and so I did. I had a few attacks over the next few weeks, but nothing as dramatic as my first experiences. This time, I was really aware of my body and what it was telling me a lot earlier than before. This condition was, to me, an eye opener to living in the moment and not wasting a second of it. I am reminded daily of the possibility of living in this ongoing state of stress, and I choose NOT to live like that, so in every moment, I choose the best option for me."

As Vanessa centered herself in her body, giving attention to the present, she was able to quiet her mind of the thoughts that caused her anxieties. She learned to release them so they would control her no longer.

Give attention to your behaviors – to all thoughts, emotions, reactions, fears, desires – as they occur in the present moment. You don't need to analyze or judge them; just observe them. Don't let them control you. When there is "stillness" in your mind, you can direct your attention toward your inner body – feel it. This doesn't mean you aren't aware of your surroundings or people around you. What you are trying to do is stay rooted in your inner body, in that stillness, and thus any outward behavior or action is transformed from a state of Doing, which is controlled by thought and fear, to a state of Being, where you see things with a different consciousness. You see the beauty, majesty and sacredness of your outer reality because you are in that state of presence.

"Life can be so simple and full of joy when there aren't so many attachments to items, people or situations and events that tie you up and don't honor you. As I remove the limiting behaviors from my life, I find I am open to new and exciting opportunities and feel that the anxiety attacks have allowed me to be more aware of the opportunities, and the pure joy and beauty in life, instead of being wound up tightly in a life with little purpose, unable to see the possibilities and wonder....

"I needed to get used to a different way of being, so now every day I begin with my morning cup of tea. The kettle is set to boil and I watch it steam up. I hear the noise of the bubbling water in the silence of the morning house. I drink earl grey or chia tea, and as I collect the tea, I take time to smell the tea leaves, and I choose a cup for the day that reflects me. As I pour the water, I hear it enter the cup and I watch as the tea becomes one with the water and the colour changes and steam rises with the aromas of the tea, all held within that moment. This is a morning ritual for me. And if I somehow miss this and find myself in the drill of the day, I can all too quickly feel a negative sensation in my body and I know intuitively that I need to come back to the moment.

"I try this process with many of the ordinary aspects of life...making dinner, watching child's play, doing the

shopping. I live with mindfulness in all that I do. This is how I live in my new and different life! My life is less cluttered with the unimportant and more full of joy, and I find time in the simplest of things. For example, one morning while having my shower, as I set the shampoo bottle down in the shower, a bubble came out of the top of the container. It wasn't a sudsy bubble; it was a clear rainbow-colored bubble and it continued to grow as I stood there. I had the thought that I must be positioned perfectly again in the right place at the right time as the shower water wasn't popping it, and I stood there admiring the amazing colours within the bubble. Then I noticed the reflection of myself surrounded by the rainbow of colours. A few years ago, I would not have even noticed that moment and it would have passed me by. I now choose to enjoy all my moments."

By living in the present moment, you can fully appreciate the moments of now. You don't mourn the past or worry about the future and anticipate troubles. This only robs you of your enjoyment of today. It robs you of truly living. If you're living in the present, you're living in acceptance of what is, realizing that everything is complete as it is. By living in the present, you have the power to change your life. You can't do this in the past; it's already happened. You can't do this in the future; it's not here yet.

To live in the present, observe your thoughts. Witness them, but don't judge them, and when your mind is still, go deep into your inner body. Practice conscious breathing in the form of meditation by focusing your attention on your breath filling your inner body. And finally, practice mindfulness by practicing awareness in all your actions, whatever they may be. See the sacredness in everything you do. That is living in the present moment!

EXERCISE

At night time, as you lie in your bed before sleep, close your eyes and go deep into your inner body. Focus on your breathing, allowing it to move in and out of your body. Feel each breath. If thoughts enter your mind, honor them and release them. Keep breathing in and out, slowly and deliberately. Then see yourself surrounded by light and breathe in this light throughout your body. Let it permeate your whole body. Just be with the feeling for as long as you need or want. You are in your inner body and experiencing the present moment.

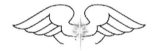

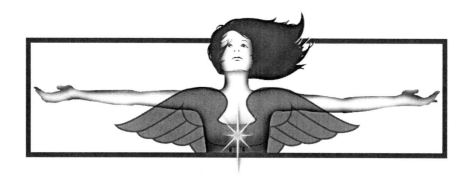

What's Really
Important in Life?

"True love and a sense of security, which we all seek, only come from within, from that heart-centered place where our god/dess essence resides. We are all part of the Divine."

I have a question for you. What do you consider important in your life? Before you were slapped upside the head by your life-altering experience, did outer material things such as your job, your title, your clothes, your house, your car or similar markers of success dictate your life? Did being recognized and admired by others mean a lot to you? What about people you encountered, including not only your family and friends but also those who came into your life at any given moment, for whatever reason? Where did they fit in your life? What about your own health and wellbeing? Did that have any bearing on how content you were with your life? Now that your life has probably taken a turn, are you content with the way it's going? If not, why?

Before my stroke, I was living a very full life, one that I thought had meaning with my corporate job, my fledgling healing arts business, and my books. I saw my corporate job as a means to an end; it was my bread and butter while I developed my healing arts business and wrote and published my books. But I actually loved my job as a corporate manager. I loved the people I worked with but, most importantly, I enjoyed the recognition I received from them for the great work I had done. Who wouldn't want the accolades I received for doing a good job? Isn't that human nature, to want acceptance from others?

I did try to balance the crazy schedule I had with some "me time," meditating every morning before work and going to the gym after, but I was on the treadmill of life, moving at a very fast speed. My two sons, with whom I have a very special relationship, seemed to be doing fine. Both were in college and my youngest was living with me, as you know. Everything seemed to be going along very smoothly – until that momentous morning when I was "brought to my knees," so to speak. It was as if I had been slapped in the face by the Divine for something displeasing. For even though I thought I was living a purposeful life, I realized that the agenda by which I was living was not in alignment with my true purpose in life. It did not agree with what was really important in my life. I should say that it wasn't my actions that didn't agree; it was my mindset and emotions behind the actions that weren't in harmony!

Let me put things into perspective, to clarify what I mean. Ever since I was young, I had lived under a cloud of anxiety – always fearful of not being able to live up to expectations of being perfect. How I compensated for that was to try to control all aspects of my life: my relationships, what I did in my life and how I did it. I didn't want to be rejected for not being perfect. When I was a ballet student, I would feign illness so I didn't have to dance if my feet hurt and I knew I wouldn't be able to perform up to par. In relationships (those after my divorce), I would always be the one to break them off because I didn't want to be rejected for not being (what I thought was) what the men wanted. At work, I would put up an invisible energy shield when I felt someone was going to ask me to do something I didn't want to do. There were limits on how much I wanted to handle and I didn't want to look like I was incapable of doing something.

Needless to say, I was in a constant state of anxiety, especially when I felt I was losing control of the situation. While my intentions of working my corporate job to pay the bills while building my business and writing books to serve others were commendable, I was functioning from the wrong mentality. My actions were a consequence of my need to live up to the expectations of others. I was basing my success in life on my outer reality, instead of what my heart spoke to me. If my actions had been heart-centered, they would have taken on a completely different essence. They would have come from an inner place of compassion and love for myself and for others – in other words, with the spirit of, "How can I serve my soul and in turn serve others?"

As I see it, if you are being guided by an open heart, success may follow or not, but it won't matter. As you are imbued with love for yourself and for others, everything else takes care of itself. If it is your destiny to be successful in your endeavors, then it will manifest because it is in perfect alignment with what the Universe wants for you. Everything is as it should be at every moment of our lives.

So, I ask the question again. What's really important in life? When you are operating from your true essence, your heart center, life takes on new meaning. No longer do outer forces run your life. No longer does your current circumstance make you who you are or who you will become. You realize that your success in life is about the relationships you have, with yourself and with others. It's about moving to that deep place within your heart from which the Divine fiber of your being resonates.

This transition to heart-based consciousness begins with you feeling unsatisfied with and uninspired by those things which used to draw your full attention. They have less meaning and purpose in your life, as they no longer provide you with the validation you need to affirm your place in the world. When your outer reality is the basis of your being, you are in a constant state of fear – fear of being alone and rejected, fear that you are no longer whole as a person because of your trauma, that you have nothing to offer – so you become defensive. You have separated yourself from the Divine; no wonder you feel alone and abandoned. True love and a sense of security, which we all seek, only come from within, from that heart-centered place where our god/dess essence resides. We are all part of the Divine.

Read below how Katherine's spiritual journey connecting with the Divine helped her move through the treacherous years of her debilitating condition to the heart-centric place of inner sanctity and love.

"In 1990, whilst in my final year at university, I had an operation to remove nasal polyps. I reacted badly to the anaesthetic and afterwards did not return to the same level of health. I knew something was wrong because I played sports that year but never got fit. With a certain level of exhaustion, I also felt low emotionally. I found this difficult and came to realize that I defined myself by having a certain level of happiness.

"I took a job after university, but 18 months later I collapsed on the way to the office. Shortly afterwards, I was finally diagnosed. The diagnosis was ME (Myalgic Encephalomyelitis), an illness now often referred to as CFS (Chronic Fatigue Syndrome) or CFIDS (Chronic Fatigue and Immune Dysfunction Syndrome).

"In 1995 I became so ill that I was completely bedbound with a commode by the bed, unable to feed myself and needing to drink through a straw. To lift a mug, place it propped up on my chest, and subdue the involuntary movements in my arms long enough to hold it was in

itself a huge endeavor. I was unable to talk much and when someone was talking to me, I found it distressing and painful to try to take in the words.

"The challenges I faced were many. The first shock was to find out that I didn't have a physical or emotional support system available. Those close to me reacted with anger to my being unable to do what I had been able to do before. I felt lonely, confused and heartbroken.

"The second major issue throughout the years of disability was an inadequate level of care. Due to reactive hypoglaecemia I needed to eat every two hours, yet, because of the muscle fatigue and pain, I could feed myself very little. With only four hours of care allocated across the day, I felt urgently hungry most of the time and struggled to keep my weight above 45 kilos (99 pounds). My chances of recovery seemed slim. I had been advised to get rest, yet the restricted care times forced me to do more than was good for me.

"In this difficult situation, I had an ongoing commitment to maintain my sense of self-worth. Sometimes we define our value by what we do. Unable to feed myself and totally dependent on others, there was no task I could carry out with ease or competence, including talking, writing or watching TV.

"It is common to define our value by what we can offer to others. In a time of illness, I did not feel I could offer much at all. (Read on to see how this view changed as the years passed by.)

"Often we define our value by the way we are perceived and treated by others. Many people contributed an amazing amount of time and effort to my care.

101

Nonetheless, I spent upwards of 20 hours a day bedbound and alone. The amount and quality of care I received often did not help to affirm my value.

"So how did I, and how can you, affirm self-worth in a time of illness? For me, spiritual beliefs, spiritual practice, spiritual experience, my relationship with Jesus, creativity and self-expression all played their part.

"I had been brought up with the spiritual belief that we are all of inherent value. I cultivated this belief through the practice of seeing the Christ in others and through the practice of forgiveness. My ability to see the value in others, along with my belief in our equality in the eyes of God, encouraged me to accept that I myself must be of value.

"The practice of forgiveness was essential to me. If you are lying still, in silence and in pain, you have only your own mind to which to listen. I developed an exercise for releasing judgement, which I practised over and over to keep bringing my mind back to a place of peace.

"Spiritual practice, including that of forgiveness, led me to experience a peace and joy that does not depend on this world, and which this world cannot give. Whenever I touched this joy, regardless of my circumstances, I was free. This experience let me know that the world of suffering is not the true reality.

"This world may push us to give up or to define our value negatively by how we are treated. Yet we can refuse to do so. We can choose to believe that we are loved by God and we are a part of love itself. And when invited to hate, we can practise love.

"In writing this, I am reminded of Jesus on the cross. He had an invitation to hate everyone who had put him there and yet he chose to love. He remembered who he was – that he was one with God. By so doing, he dropped the illusion of the body and rose again, showing that there is no death.

"I had been brought up Catholic and had left the church at 17 because I was so grief-stricken by the crucifixion. Early on in the illness, I came across the book A Course in Miracles. A Course in Miracles, *along with other books including those by Christian authors, helped me question and heal my relationship with Jesus. To receive love, guidance and healing from Jesus has been another part of my journey to be defined other than by the world. I am a follower of Jesus and feel immense love for him. His journey has been a huge example to me throughout the years of illness.*

"In this chapter I use the term 'self-worth,' yet, in many ways, my journey has been one of shifting from self-worth to knowing my worth through my spiritual identity as part of God and as one in Christ. It is a seeming paradox that as we drop the 'self,' self-worth naturally results – a sense of worth which flows not from what we do but from the knowledge of our existence as part of All That Is. We are part of the love, the joy, the peace, which we know experientially to be of inherent value. I believe that in the end, this is our only value.

"Other important factors in finding value and life within the experience of illness were creativity and self-expression.

"I lived in a world where I had little to reflect back to me who I was. In the first years off work, I was housebound and saw few people. Once I was bedbound, I mainly

saw strangers – caregivers – with no knowledge of who I had been prior to illness, and with little ability to get to know me due to my minimal speech. My writing served the purpose of giving me a sense of being known and understood, even if only by myself.

"*In the early days of illness, I wrote a great deal. In 1995, the muscle fatigue spread from my legs to include my arms and I could no longer write normally. (One might have argued that I shouldn't have been writing at all, as I needed my arms to feed myself as much as I could. But without some form of expression, the intense loneliness, heartbreak and fear would have led me to give up.)*

"*A few years later someone gave me a dictaphone, someone else found me a typist, and my life changed. When I was alone, I could speak more easily, with as many breaks as I needed. I could now dictate what was in my mind.*

"*Around 1994, I read* The Celestine Prophecy *by James Redfield. It includes the interesting proposition that our questions are just as important as our answers. If there is a source of wisdom available to us, we can form a question, relax into a place of trust, and the answer will be given.*

"*An extraordinary adventure started. I would ask questions and, to my surprise, entire poems would form in my head.*

"*I experienced my writing as guidance from God – the answers to my questions. Over the years, I dictated around 6,000 poems and developed a system of self-talk. Bit by bit, I am now editing and publishing these writings to form travel guides on the psycho-spiritual journey. My prayer and my experience is that they serve others in the same way they served (and continue to serve) me.*

"In 2008, after 14 years of being bedbound, I experienced dramatic healing that brought me to a place of being able to walk and talk again. My life still involves managing the condition of ME/CFS. Nonetheless, it is a rich and wonderful life. Every day I work on writing books to continue my own journey, and to share what I have learned of finding peace in a difficult situation whatever the difficulty may be. Likewise, I run a successful website on spirituality and healing. And at times I give poetry readings and talks from my books. Most importantly, I touch the peace and joy of reality throughout each day.

"Despite once more being active in the world, I am convinced that our most profound service to ourselves and to the world is the extent to which we are willing to open our minds and hearts to receive God's love. A time of difficulty brings to our awareness the ways in which we block out that love; it invites us to allow God to remove these blocks and love us just as we are. As we do so, we also allow love to flow more easily into the lives of others. I know of many beautiful people living with illness and difficulties who provide this valuable service to us all. If you are one of them, you truly are a radiant survivor."

As you can see from Katherine's story, as she sought to find out who she was beyond her illness through her connection with the Creator, she was able to journey down the path of her long recovery to that place of inner peace and love, and share what she learned with others.

If you are seeking love and security from outside yourself, feeding on outside energies, you are turning your attention away from yourself. Your self-worth becomes rooted in the outer world's judgments of your outside appearance, not your true inner being. Thus, you feel you have to "control" your actions, your behaviors, and your personality, so that you are accepted in the world.

But what if you were to surrender that control and turn inward to accept yourself – the inner self – the center of your true personal power, with all its self-love, self-admiration and a soul level of security? When you are working from this heart-centered place of self-love and self-awareness, you no longer need approval from the outside. You free yourself from all outer attachments. By no longer spending all your energy on controlling your thoughts and behavior to accommodate the opinions of others, you can create an open space from which your Divine power can radiate within, and then beam its immense light outwardly into the world. You feel liberated. You begin to feel at peace with yourself as you are. And when you are content with who you are, you begin to feel compassion for others, for who they are just as themselves. There is no judgment about who they "should be." And instead of your actions and behavior being directed by the "what's in it for me?" mindset, they become "they" oriented. Ultimately, we are all put on this earth to help each other. We cannot accomplish anything in this world alone.

As with Katherine, my recovery from my stroke encompassed many lessons, one of them being that I needed to move to a heart-based consciousness. I do hope that as you evaluate your life, you come to the same conclusion of what's really important in life: that beautiful relationship you have with yourself, which will serve as a beacon of light that will brighten the path of others as they follow their own personal journey.

EXERCISE

In your journal or notebook, write down what's really important to you in life and what ways you can strive to do those things that are important. What brings you to that heart-centric consciousness?

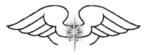

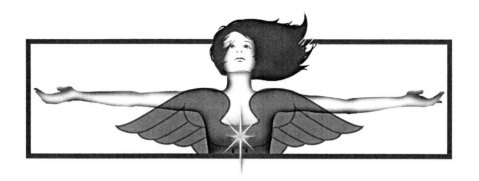

Recovery Is a Process

"Know that you will go through some or all of the stages of recovery, as it is necessary to deal with any emotions that are triggered as you walk the path to your new life."

E verything in life is a process. Life itself is a process. We begin our physical life as an infant. We then evolve into a toddler, a child, adolescent, teenager, young adult and adult, experiencing all the nuances of each stage, and the process continues until our physical body dies. And if you believe in reincarnation, the process starts all over again in another incarnation, over and over until you are no longer in a physical form.

As a human being who has faced some sort of trauma in your life, you will experience the process of recovery as you travel down the path of rehabilitation that leads you to the awakening of a new life. The most well-known process of recovery is that of Elisabeth Kübler-Ross, who introduced her hypothesis of "the five stages of grief" in her book *On Death and Dying.* Although this hypothesis is about the emotions one goes through when one is grieving the loss of a loved one, it embraces any sort of life-threatening or life-altering event in one's life. It is not meant to be a complete account of all the possible emotions a person could feel when he or she is challenged by trauma. Nor will everyone experience all five stages, or even in the order in which she has defined them, as we are all unique individuals with our own individual recovery adventures. These five stages of grief (which we will call "stages of recovery" for the purposes of this book) are: denial, anger, bargaining, depression and acceptance. See how they've played a role in your journey of recovery.

Denial is a defense mechanism used when a person is unable to face the reality of a situation. He or she "turns a blind eye," so to speak. Life makes no sense anymore. You ask yourself how you can go on or why you should continue to live. Usually, a person tries to find ways just to get through each day. But it can require a lot of psychic energy to maintain such a state. The grace of denial, though, is that nature uses it as a way to let in only as much as a person can handle. And as you start to accept reality, you initiate the healing process, where all the feelings you are denying begin to surface.

Anger is usually the most prominent feeling you will have. You start asking questions like, "Why did this happen?" or, "Why did God let this happen?" Other emotions usually surface from beneath the anger, especially pain, but anger is the one we normally contend with first. And your anger may have no boundaries, since it may extend to your friends, your family, your doctors, God or anyone else close to you.

Then you may start bargaining with God, wishing and begging for life to return to the way it was. You may get lost in a maze of "what if" or "if only" statements where guilt becomes your companion. *What could I have done differently to prevent the trauma?* You may remain in the past to avoid the ensuing pain of the present.

Then depression sets in as you move from the past to the present, knowing you can't go back to what was. You experience very deep levels of grief and pain, and feel that it's going to last forever. You may withdraw from life, wondering if you really want to go on living. Depression is a normal feeling when faced with trauma, and a necessary stop along the road to recovery.

But then you realize you have a new reality and slowly begin to accept it as your present day life. It doesn't mean you feel okay about it, or that you like this reality, but eventually you see it as your new existence and learn to live with it. It becomes your new norm. And slowly but surely, you can begin to enjoy life again, making the necessary changes to accommodate your circumstances. You start making new connections as old ones fall away. You don't deny your feelings any longer; instead, you listen to your needs. You change and evolve as you start reaching out to others and become more involved with life. You start to see what's really important in life. Life becomes joyous again.

When I had my stroke and the few weeks following, I was oblivious to my condition. I knew I was bedridden. I went to my inpatient rehab religiously. I regularly woke up in the wee hours of the morning for the nurses to draw blood, since I was on Coumadin (a blood thinner), which needed to be monitored. I wandered the halls in my wheelchair, talking to the nurses and other patients. But it didn't really hit me that my life had drastically changed. It was like a blip on the radar screen. Perhaps that was my denial, my way of coping with what had happened. I don't think I ever really got angry or tried to bargain with God about my situation, since I saw it as my karma, my way of reconciling my past, as I explained in "My Story." Any depression that I felt came in the form of severe anxiety disorder that lasted for about a month, three months following my stroke. I was so relieved when it finally let up because I felt like I was living in hell. I even became a bit suicidal – not that I would ever take my life, but the thought did cross my mind a few times when I was in the throes of the anxiety.

Overall, I had little problem accepting my condition because of my beliefs of why, on a spiritual level, I'd had my stroke. Embracing this viewpoint carried me through the journey. Of course, there were days of sadness and impatience and questioning whether I would ever get better; but by heeding everything I've talked about in this book, I was able to travel the long and difficult road with spirits lifted high most of the time. And the further along the road to recovery I got, the more confident I became that full recovery was only a matter of time and patience. As I said before, I hoped I would be fully recovered by the time I finished this book, but if not, I wouldn't be far off.

I would now like to share Joe's story of sexual abuse by a priest when he was young and his process of recovery.

"My childhood unofficially ended in June 1980. I was a few months short of my 11th birthday, but the innocence that most kids get to experience was stolen from me.

"I was the kid who didn't even fit in with the rest of the misfits in school. I was too intelligent for my own good, and yet I had no common sense and no social skills. I trusted too easily, was not very streetwise, and I was starved for attention. My father had a great job, but it involved a lot of shift work...not an ideal condition for building a solid, healthy relationship. My mother did the best she could, but it just wasn't enough. (I should add that my younger sister and brother turned out just fine.) I was the perfect target for a pedophile.

"In January 1980, a new priest was transferred to the Catholic Church we attended. He was very charismatic and enthusiastic, and since he was so much younger than the other two priests, he was placed in charge of the altar boy program. My mother was quite taken by him. She had the idea that since my father's schedule was the way it was, maybe this priest could be the male role model I needed. My father, on the other hand, wasn't as impressed. He felt that something was 'a little

off' and didn't trust him the way my mother did. He also didn't like the modern touches this priest brought to Mass (singing the prayers, using incense, etc.). But he decided to leave decisions like this to my mother.

"So, in June 1980, with her blessing, I went on an overnight trip to the priest's family cabin about a 90-minute drive from my house. He cooked dinner while I watched a baseball game, and after dinner (and a beer or two), he put on one of the movies he'd rented. I can assure you, it wasn't The Muppet Movie.

"This was my first exposure to sex in any form. At the age of 10. With a 40-something-year-old priest. First a movie, then a 'hands-on' demonstration. I won't go into specific details about what he did or made me do, but suffice to say that no 10-year-old should have to go through what I endured. What I will say is that each time, when he was 'done with me' (for lack of a better term), he would shuffle me off to my own bedroom and leave me alone with my thoughts. I felt ashamed, used and abandoned. But I was so desperate for the attention that I tucked those feelings aside.

"As he drove me home the next afternoon, he made me promise not to tell anyone about anything that happened in that cabin. He claimed to have the authority to send me to Hell and have my family kicked out of the church if I did say anything. Of course, I didn't tell anyone.

"There was one fall visit when I came home with a hickey on my collarbone. I tried to keep it covered up, but my father noticed it one day. When he asked about it, I told him I had been doing yard work and a tree branch had hit me. I knew he didn't believe me, but how could I tell him the truth? I was too scared.

"After around 50 overnight stays during the next 7 years, I managed to end it the summer after my high school graduation. During the last trip up there, I made up a story about having a girlfriend...and I felt guilty for lying to a priest. That's pretty sick.

"I survived by blocking it all out, burying it, repressing those memories...but the after-effects remained. When I went in the Navy, I rebelled. I didn't want to be there. I joined because my father had served for eight years and I thought I could impress him by following in his footsteps. I signed up for six years, but got kicked out after three years, two months and five days. He wasn't impressed.

"Within the span of three weeks in June 1988, I failed my Navy school, was dumped by my girlfriend, and found out my parents were getting divorced. I gave up on everything and decided to kill myself (twice without success...talk about feeling like a failure).

"I was assigned to a ship based in Norfolk, Virginia. I really didn't want to be there. The thrill of seeing the world was gone. I went AWOL a couple times...then I decided to go back home to Illinois for Christmas. What I didn't know at the time was that people like me almost always try to return home for the holidays. They had a BOLO (be on lookout) for me and my car. When I pulled off the highway to get gas and a soda, they were waiting and I was arrested ten minutes from my mother's apartment. On Christmas Eve. I ended up spending four months in prison for desertion.

"The Navy determined that I had a drinking problem, which contributed to my lack of discipline. They sent me to rehab and I was forced to attend recovery meetings, which bored me to tears. I wasn't ready or willing to do

anything. Even if I hadn't repressed the memories of my abuse, I was in absolutely no condition to take any steps to solve my problems.

"I drank my way out of the Navy. I was discharged 3 months after I turned 21 and I quit drinking a couple months later. I decided to go back to the recovery meetings and started doing what I was supposed to do (for once). I got to the point where I almost felt as if my life was getting better.

"One night, out of the blue, my roommate asked me if I had been sexually abused as a kid. All the memories flooded back and I broke down in tears as I said that I had. I found a support group and a counselor and tried to deal with it as best I could. I hired an attorney and filed a civil suit against the priest, the bishop in charge of the diocese, and the diocese itself. Unfortunately, the criminal statute of limitations had expired the day I turned 20.

"Against the advice of many people, I decided to use my name when I filed my lawsuit. As my attorney started working on my case, he discovered that I was one of more than 70 victims from 3 different churches in the diocese. There were police reports filed against the priest at his previous parish, but they somehow disappeared just before he was reassigned to mine.

"I was angry (and for good reason). I had given up on God, faith, church, all of it, years earlier. I found myself questioning how a loving God could allow something like this to happen to one of His children. I used to say, halfjokingly, that if I ever set foot in a church again, it would probably collapse around me. I had given up on society. I saw no redeeming qualities in a world that allowed this sort of tragedy to go on. I had given up on myself, too. I

had become cold and cynical and felt unworthy of any love.

"I knew I needed some help. I started seeing a counselor, bought myself a teddy bear (yes, at 24), and began the process of healing. I eventually realized that my recovery had actually started when I answered that question three years earlier: yes, I was sexually abused as a child. I eventually found a support group consisting of men and women who had answered that same question and had also stepped onto that road to healing.

"The leader of our group was a priest who had been sexually abused as a child. He encouraged me to speak out and not be afraid of what anyone might say to me or about me. Because of him, I found the strength and courage to get involved in an HBO special called 'Priestly Sins.' I watched it again a few years ago and was amazed that I actually did it.

"I have slowly, gradually, grown into a real adult. I've gone from three or four jobs in one year to [holding down] one job...for over eight years. I've gone from bouncing around the country to living in the same house for over nine years. I've gone from a string of failed relationships to being with an amazing woman for close to ten years. I am as stable and happy as I can ever remember being.

"Don't get me wrong. Life is far from perfect. Some days it's still downright uncomfortable. A part of me still wishes I had never gone through that horrendous experience. I still have to live in my own skin, listening to the thoughts rattle around in my brain. But I always hear a voice that reminds me that if I hadn't, I wouldn't be where I am today. The difference is that now I know my past does not define me. The difference is that now

my emotions aren't ruling me. The difference is that I'm no longer ashamed.

"The biggest difference, however, is that I have started to rebuild my relationship with God. I've stopped asking Him why it happened. Instead, I am asking what good I can do because it happened. I found a church that focuses on the Word of God instead of the word of man, a church that has adopted the slogan 'No Perfect People Allowed' and welcomed me regardless of my faults and my past. I chose to be baptized and have committed myself to living a better life.

"There have been a lot of people who unknowingly helped me recover and grow. People who just listened to me vent, cry, scream, complain, and question everything. People who said what I needed to hear, as opposed to what I wanted to hear. People who let me make mistakes and, instead of belittling me for them, showed me how to grow and learn from them. People who knew how to help me not only sort out my feelings, but show me how to turn them into something constructive. People who helped me find the good in myself. People who thanked me for being so brave and courageous. People whose bravery and courage I held up as an example.

"My case helped expose the massive cover-up in the church. Dozens of priests had been clandestinely transferred from parish to parish because of allegations against them. The parents of these children were stonewalled and flat-out lied to by the church hierarchy. Many people came forward and admitted that they, too, were victims. The criminal statute of limitations in Illinois was also re-examined and eventually changed. The period of time to file criminal charges was extended from 2 years to 20 years (after the child victim turned 20).

"Recovering has been a long, enlightening, and sometimes painful process. But I have to say that every step has been worth it. And yes, I still have that teddy bear."

As you can see, Joe went through the different stages in his own unique way. He experienced denial when he repressed the memories. And his anger showed up in the Navy when he rebelled because he didn't want to be there, and when he started to question "how a loving God could allow something like this to happen to one of His children." He may have tried to use drinking as his way of bargaining, since we will do anything during this phase to avoid the pain. Depression set in when his life seemed worthless and he tried to kill himself twice. Finally, he accepted that he needed help and went into individual and group counseling to help him through the healing process.

Recovery IS a process, which can take days, weeks, months, years or a lifetime, depending on how traumatic the situation is. Know that you will go through some or all of the stages of recovery, as it is necessary to deal with any emotions that are triggered as you walk the path to your new life. And when you have reached that place of acceptance and see that new life ahead of you, may you rejoice in your victory as a survivor and a thriver!

EXERCISE

In your journal or notebook, write down how you have gone through (or are going through) your recovery process. Which phases have you gone through? Where are you now? What emotions have come up in each phase? What can you do or are you doing to ease the process along, understanding that there are some things you can change and some you can't, no matter how hard things seem to be? It helps in your recovery to know what phases you go through and how you can make your recovery as easy as possible, accepting the challenges and moving through them with strength and conviction.

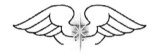

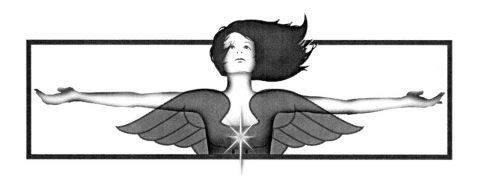

What if I Don't
Fully Recover?

"Know that only you can dictate what your life will become after trauma...there's nothing you can't do in your life!"

What will life be like if I don't fully recover? That's a very valid question to ask when you're in the midst of a life trauma. You may have just experienced your ordeal, or you may have struggled for so long with your condition that maybe you see progress or maybe you don't, and you may ask yourself, "Am I always going to have to live this way?"

I have fallen into this mindset, even though everyone and everything has indicated that I would fully recover and actually be better than I was before, as I've mentioned. But that nasty little thing we call "fear," which hides deep in one's psyche until just the right time to jump out and surprise us, came up from behind and grabbed me. Overcoming one's fears does take time, especially if those fears are deeply rooted. Let me tell you about another time when this inner fear was triggered.

It was the second week in January 2013. It was supposed to be a new era of transformation and I felt it was just that, as I was beginning to feel my body getting stronger. The muscles on my paralyzed side were coming back to life because the nerves were finally beginning to function again, innervating the muscles. Where before my leg and arm just felt "floppy" when fatigued or overworked, now I could "feel the burn" as Jane Fonda would say in her workout DVDs. My right side (my paralyzed side) began to feel more normal and I was elated. In rehab of that second week, my therapist was impressed at my progress even since the week before, when he told me I needed to believe in myself.

And then I came down with the flu, which completely incapacitated me. From one day to the next, I went from being on top of the world, flying high with delight at my progress, to falling deep into the pit of agony and seeming decline. Every ounce of strength I had was zapped and my body, or should I say half my body, felt stiff, mechanical and unyielding. I certainly couldn't walk or use my arm with the same grace I had when I was a ballet dancer many, many moons ago. As stiff as my body felt, I began to think I would always be that way and I had better accept it.

I remembered what the Body Talk System[26] practitioner I went to for several months once asked me: "Can you accept it if you remain as you are, always? If you can, you can realize that your life isn't about your situation. You can move forward with life as it is."

I started thinking about this statement and, to my surprise, I was able to accept that as a possible truth for me. I may not fully recover and I'm okay with that. Yeah, I wanted to get back to my salsa lessons and I wanted to have love in my life again and I wanted to live on my own again, but the fact of the matter was that I was able to accept me just as I was at that moment. And you know what happened because of my acknowledgment? My fear of not being able to recover fully went away and my body started responding again, even though I hadn't been able to do any rehab or exercise for a week. I was back on my road to full recovery.

But what happens if you truly won't recover fully from your trauma? The story below was taken from Sue's website Lifegeta.co.uk, with her permission. It's a tale of tragedy and triumph in which Sue shows how you can take a seemingly impossible situation and turn it into a personal victory, and then take it and make it into a beacon of light for many others. She didn't let her disability stop her from living a full, happy life.

"On April 24, 1993, at the age of 26 I had 2 major strokes that changed my life dramatically. Life before my stroke was a mix of a glamorous day job working for a 'high-end' cosmetics company in London, and working and socializing at a nightclub.

"The week before my stroke I had been to aerobics on Sunday as normal. (I'm not particularly sporty, just doing it to get a bit healthy at the time!) For the next week I had a pain in the neck (sorry about the pun!). It hurt if I turned quickly, but I just assumed that I had done it at aerobics.

"The night before my stroke I settled down to do some paperwork that I'd brought home from work, had a glass of wine, painted my nails, and then bed. I remember getting up for a drink of water and feeling fine.

"The next morning I remember feeling a little faint as I bent over the sink to clean my teeth, so I sat on the loo hoping the feeling would pass. (I remember thinking, I'm never going to drink wine again when I have to be up for work in the morning!) Then I felt as if my left side was melting. There was no pain, just a feeling that everything was in slow motion. Somehow I managed to stagger back into the bedroom (so I could walk then!). As I lay on the bed, the feeling seemed to be growing. Soon I

had pins and needles on the whole of my left-hand side, but there was still no pain as I recall.

"*I had just had a phone extension put in, so I was able to call for help. My movements were slow and I found it hard to dial the numbers. I know it sounds a bit morbid but I truly believe that if I hadn't had the phone in the bedroom, I wouldn't be here today, as I would not have been able to get down the stairs. I tried to call my mum and when she answered, I found that I could hardly speak. I managed to get out the words 'Mum' and 'I don't feel right' but then I dropped the phone. She arrived about 10 minutes later. I started to vomit and continued to be ill like this every 10 minutes or so. When my GP arrived, he did a few reflex tests and called an ambulance to take me to the local hospital, but I don't remember the trip.*

"*At the hospital, I was taken to A&E and it was at this point I heard the word 'stroke' (CVA or cardio vascular accident). I remember thinking, I can't have had a stroke. I'm only 26! That's what old people have! Boy, was I in for an eye opener! I was taken by ambulance to the hospital in London to have a CT scan to see what the problem was exactly. Once the scan was done, I was wheeled to a small consulting room to wait for the results. However, the doctor said they were inconclusive and he would like to keep me in for a couple days.*

"*Once on the ward, I started to feel strange again, as if everything was in slow motion. I remember giggling because I had a big snot bubble and I couldn't seem to coordinate my arm to get rid of it (sorry for the description, but I don't know how else to put it). I recall a nurse coming into my cubicle, but after that I don't remember anything. That was when I had stroke number 2! The BIGGIE (knocked out my whole right side, my breathing, gag reflex...well everything, just about!) I woke up about 24 hours later in intensive care and felt like I was in a straitjacket, strapped to the bed. Then I realized the reason I felt like this was because I was paralyzed from the neck down.*

"The nurse came in and explained that I was unable to speak because I had lost my gag reflex (unable to swallow); therefore, my voice box was not working either. I knew what I wanted to say, but no sound would come out, even though I was able to 'mouth' words. I was surrounded by lots of machines. There was a ventilator, as I was unable to breathe unaided, and I also had a Nassau-gastric tube and there were pads on my chest checking my vital signs, as well as drips in my arms and neck. The nurse told me not to worry about the loo, as I had a catheter fitted. I remember feeling like a baby, not being able to speak, move or even control my own bowel movements.

"A doctor came round to see me and told me I had suffered another suspected stroke whilst I was on the ward. This had been more severe and was the reason I had lost consciousness. The stroke I had in the morning affected my left side and the one I had in hospital affected my right side. This ward was to become my home for the next 12 weeks, although I didn't realize that at the time! I thought what had happened to me would right itself soon and that I would be back to 'normal' (whatever that is!).

"I started having physiotherapy quite soon after being admitted to ICU. Just getting me out of bed and sitting me in a chair was a long drawn-out job needing about three therapists and a hoist, as I was like a rag doll. The

physiotherapy I was having was passive. So many things were happening to me, I felt so out of control and I could see people I cared for getting upset (with happy faces, but their eyes told a different story). I felt there was nothing I could do to comfort them.

"*During this time, I also had an MRI scan. The results showed that I had split the two main carotid arteries in my neck. They had ruptured on both sides; that's why I couldn't move my left or right side. The damage was mainly in the lower brain stem (which acts like the body's supervisor, telling the messages from the brain where to go, or what to move, like your leg or your arm).*

"*The feeling in my left side came back slowly; it started with my hand and gradually, over a period of days, I was able to move my fingers again; and finally I could move my arm a bit. My left leg was also getting stronger and I was able to move it slightly. My left leg and arm had been still for so long that when I started to get movement in them, I got awful cramps. Although they hurt, I was glad to feel something, even pain! About this time I had to have another scan called an angiogram. The conclusion of this was that the bleed from the two carotid arteries in my neck seemed to be healing, so no need for surgery (phew!) and there was no other sign of any of my other arteries splitting or any further abnormalities. This was good, since surgery was the last option, as the part of my artery that was affected was near my brain stem and operating would have been dangerous!*

"*By this time, the tube in my mouth was making my throat ulcerated, and as I still couldn't breathe, eat or talk yet, it was decided that I would have to have a tracheotomy (an air tube fitted through a hole in my throat connected to my windpipe). When I had it fitted a few days later, I felt quite relieved to have the pipe out of my mouth. It made 'mouthing' words easier!*

"The doctors started talking about transferring me to another hospital for further treatment. I spent the next three months at St Thomas' in London, getting weaned off my ventilator. This was my first view of life as a person with a disability and, to be honest, it scared the hell out of me! The last three months I had been in intensive care, in bed most of the time, in one room. I know this might sound strange but because I had only used a wheelchair a handful of times and I didn't associate my inability to 'walk' with needing to use a wheelchair to get around, I was still thinking as though I 'could' walk!

"Gradually after about three months, I started to breathe for myself and eat, so my tracheotomy and feeding tube were removed. And my double vision had improved, but had not gone completely.

"It was felt that I needed to go to a rehabilitation unit to prepare me for my 'new' life as a person in a wheelchair! So the next six months were spent in a rehab unit at Addenbrooks Hospital in Cambridge. In total, I went to three hospitals and was 'in' for 52 weeks! I received physiotherapy for the entire year and still nothing! I still couldn't walk.

"I sank into a deep depression! I was 28 in a wheelchair, no job and I'd put on 2 stone (28 pounds) in weight. I started to drink to forget (I was never an alcoholic or anything, it's just while I felt 'tipsy' I could pretend I was okay again!). Then I fell out of my wheelchair and caught my head on the corner of the table, causing a nasty gash on my eyelid!

"As I waited in Casualty, I realized it was up to me to change my life. I could go on feeling sorry for myself or I could give myself a 'kick up the bum' and stop looking for someone else to blame. I started taking my physiotherapy seriously, put myself on a good healthy eating plan and stopped drinking alcohol. I lost weight sensibly, and I was able put my electric chair away. Using my manual chair to get around helped me become more active. Then I began to try and take a few steps, walking with the aid of a stick and a few well-placed grab rails around my flat. I can walk a little outside but still use my chair for longer distances, but I'm sure that with time and a positive attitude I'll get back even more mobility."

The above story was written about five years after Sue's stroke. Since then, she has taken her circumstances to new heights. She has become a life coach and mentor, founding the organization Lifegeta, which is a peer-to-peer group addressing the emotional needs of those whose bodies don't work the way they used to because of an acquired disability (i.e. stroke, head injury, etc.) or diagnosis (i.e. MS, Parkinson's, etc.). Her group work includes discussion groups, monthly meetings, workshops, self-development courses and the like. Her work is to help others adapt to their new lives as disabled persons, to help lift them from the depression they may feel into a realm filled with hope for a new future.

Sue has also been on radio programs, has done speaking engagements where she and Lifegeta have received awards from stroke organizations, and she has visited the British House of Lords. She has also swum with dolphins, made a trip to Singapore, and even had a Caribbean cruise right in the comfort of her own flat. Since she couldn't go to the Caribbean, she brought the Caribbean to her. Donned in her brown tankini and shorts, she cranked up the heat in her flat and lay back, comfy in a lounge chair surrounded by magazines and a rubber ring, listening to calypso music and sipping exotic drinks with a blow-up palm tree standing like a sentinel over her. "I know there's nothing I can't do if I set my mind to it. After all, if I can manage a living room cruise, I can do most anything."

"There IS life after _____. I'm living proof of it!" Fill in the blank with your circumstance. Know that only you can dictate what your life will become after trauma. By heeding all that has been said in the chapters of this book, there's nothing you can't do in your life. Never give up and always believe in yourself. Don't let limiting beliefs stop you from being all you can be. Be grateful for what you have and keep an uplifted attitude, even in moments of despair. Know you have all the support you need through family, friends and your own inner divinity. You can either rise to the occasion or you can fall into the darkness of the soul and never get back up. It's your choice! Wouldn't you rather shine and thrive as a survivor and victor?

EXERCISE

In your journal or notebook, write down the things you used to do in the left column, and then the things you can do now in your new life in the right column. Your life may have changed dramatically, but that doesn't mean it can't be just as rewarding and fulfilling. It may just be different. Find things that will challenge and fulfill you as you take on your future with zeal.

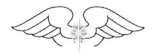

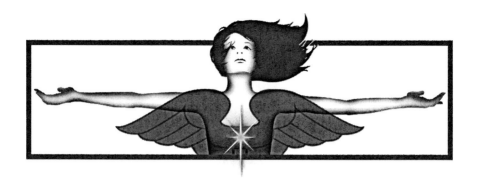

You Can
Survive and Thrive

"By bringing yourself back to your heart center, to that place of inner peace and abundance, the fear imposed by your difficulties in your outer reality is superseded by the knowledge that all is as it should be, and by having faith that there will be a positive outcome."

Have you ever been in a situation where you thought it was the end of the world, that there was no solution to your issue, that it would be your downfall? (Okay, I may be exaggerating a little, but I used to be this way sometimes, since I can be very emotional and I would let my anxieties get the better of me. I would become like Chicken Little telling everyone, "Oh, the sky is falling!") Now, I'm not talking about the condition you're trying to recover from. What I'm talking about is another life situation you may be facing on top of that. You may think, *After all I've been through with my ordeal, now I have to contend with yet another crisis?* Sometimes, when it rains, it pours.

My crisis came in the way of finances. Granted, financial difficulties may not seem a big deal considering what you've been through, but they had always plagued me, causing great anxiety throughout my adult life, and who needs to be faced with additional stress, to add to the already dire circumstances of one's life? What I wish to show is how we have the wherewithal to survive and thrive in our situations no matter how serious they may be, through our sense of inner guidance and positivity.

First, let me provide a little background. As I said, I had always struggled with money. I'm sure some of you have had the same struggles at some time in your life, or possibly even now. I think I was plagued with "bad money karma." For me, it's twofold. There were those times when it was a sincere struggle. And there were those times when it was due to my impulsiveness. Well, one of my biggest sincere struggles was when I got divorced. I tried to go out on my own as a massage therapist. I was trying to get out of being a corporate cog and do what I was passionate about (being in the healing arts), but I struggled for several years; it took time to build clientele and make the money needed to sustain me and my two young sons.

Over the course of five years, I was on unemployment three times and since I couldn't always pay my bills, I used my credit cards. Needless to say, I got myself in a huge bind with the credit card companies. My saving grace was my mom and my brother. My mom subsidized what I owed on my credit cards by refinancing her house, as it was a sizable chunk of change that I owed. (My mom is an angel!) It has taken me years to pay her back.

Well, my financial saga hadn't ended as I began writing this chapter, especially because I was on disability and only made half of what I was making before my stroke. I was barely able to make ends meet. Then several new expenses came into play and, as usual, being awakened in the middle of the night by nature and my monkey mind, I started wondering where the heck I was going to get the money to pay for everything. I had no savings to speak of and I had very little in my retirement fund.

My financial karma needed some work, since I'd always struggled. I guess this was part of my "sacred contract" with the Divine (see "You Knew Your Trauma before You Were Born") and I had to work through my financial karma in this lifetime. And since we're in the era of transformation in our world, both on a microcosmic and macrocosmic level, why wouldn't this be one of those shifts I had to make? It would all tie nicely with the big changes I was making because of my stroke, specifically moving from that ego-based mindset to being more heart-centered.

Remember that the ego is focused on one's outer reality, including the material things one has. By bringing yourself back to your heart center, to that place of inner peace and abundance, the fear imposed by your difficulties in your outer reality is superseded by the knowledge that all is as it should be, and by having faith that there will be a positive outcome. Sometimes in the past, when I had been faced with having more bills than money to pay for them, somehow some money had shown up at just the right moment. This was another one of those moments. I realized I had nothing to fear, and by believing in a positive outcome, Spirit would present the resources that would help me attain what I needed. And maybe one day, I would be free of my financial karma!

With that knowledge that all is as it should be, and by seeking your Divine inner guidance and positivity, you will acquire an inner abundance that will permeate your life in all ways: emotionally, physically, mentally and spiritually.

The story I wish to share with you is about a woman whose positive beliefs allowed her to realize that inner abundance, in spite of the serious challenges she faced in her life. Sabine was born with no arms to speak of. And then in 2012, she had a stroke.

"I was born in 1962 in Germany to two wonderful human beings. When Mom was pregnant with me, she took the drug Thalidomide to ward off the nausea and

insomnia that so often accompanies pregnancy. But what the doctors didn't know was that the medication caused birth defects in the unborn child. Thus, I was born with missing arms. But my deformity didn't stop my parents from loving me any less.

"When I was nine months old, Mom took me to physiotherapy to begin to learn how to use my feet and legs as my hands and arms. As I grew older, I learned to dress myself, comb my hair, cook, write, sew, even drive a car...just about anything a person with arms could do. And when I had my son, I learned how to feed him as an infant and to care for him as he grew older.

"Although I was able to do most tasks of raising my son, there were certain ones that I got help with. My son was born in France and, because of my disability, the country's government arranged for me to have an assistant who came twice a week to help me. She bathed him and cooked his food, putting it in small containers and freezing it. Other tasks like dressing him and carrying him were also very difficult, but I managed. This is because my parents raised me to believe in myself, telling me I can do anything I want to do. It was their positive upbringing that has gotten me through all the challenges of my life.

"But they were also very hard on my brother and me. If we wanted something, we had to earn it. I had my first job at 16 in an old folks' home, serving as a companion to the residents there, listening to their stories and just being with them, keeping them company. This experience planted the seed in me of wanting to help others. My parents also felt that education was important, so I got a Bachelor's Degree in Social Work, a Master's in Psychology and I'm now also a licensed Real

Estate Agent serving New Mexico and Colorado. And I have traveled throughout the United States and Europe as a motivational speaker, trying to dispel misconceptions and prejudices about disabilities. My motto is: 'With courage, strength, perseverance, innovative thinking and spirit, we can handle challenging life circumstances and even become stronger human beings.'

"I've had a lot of challenges in my life, but I can't and won't let them dampen my spirit. In 1995, the father of my son died of a brain aneurysm. In 1996, my fiancé died in a motorcycle accident. In 2005, my son was diagnosed with a rare case of leukemia, at the age of 21. But after three-and-a-half years of chemotherapy and fighting the cancer, he came out it. He is now 29 years old, is cancer-free and going to be a daddy in April 2013. Miracles do happen!

"Then in May 2012, I had a stroke. A friend and I were on our way to the D. H. Lawrence Ranch in Taos, New Mexico, when it happened. As I was driving, it became a very precarious situation, to say the least. Fortunately, my friend took control of the car wheel and prevented us from crashing. When I got to the hospital, they administered a medicine called tPA to break up the blood clot that had caused me to have a stroke. I was paralyzed on my left side, which was no small feat to overcome, considering I was left-handed and I only had tiny arms (three inches long). Even though I do have small appendages, I did eat with my hands. But now I had to learn how to do it with my right hand.

"I was in rehabilitation for three weeks, followed by five-and-a-half months of outpatient therapy. I also had a home program that I followed and continue to follow, to *strengthen my left side. I'm about 80% recovered in my writing ability. I have to write slowly, but it is legible again. One thing that was scary for me was learning how to drive again, since I was driving when I had my stroke. If it weren't for my friend being in the car, I wouldn't be here today.*

"Since my stroke, I have written five motivational speeches that I have given throughout New Mexico. I am moving to San Diego in March 2013, and when I do, I hope to reach a broader audience, getting involved with stroke associations and holding fundraisers for disability organizations. I was doing this before I had my stroke and I want to continue my efforts.

"I always believed I could make it, always convinced that I could do everything even when I would sometimes wonder, 'Why did this happen to me?' But I always thought I would survive. My parents really instilled this in me in a big way. I have to thank them from the bottom of my heart for having faith in me and encouraging me to be the very best I could be, in spite of my challenges.

"When I was in rehab, I would always say to myself, 'Yes, you can.' When I had trouble with my paralyzed leg, I would visualize my left foot threading a needle and tell myself that my foot could move a little, and within 45 minutes to an hour, it would start moving slightly. I went from being able to pick up a cotton ball to picking up a pencil to picking up a tube of Chapstick, which is small and more difficult to pick up. Then I returned to my writing. I will always have a 'can do' attitude. Life can be pretty harsh sometimes, but with an attitude of 'yes' instead of 'no,' you can do anything and be anything you want to become."

There's something to be said about having the right attitude. It can carry you through the thickest fog, where you can't see where you're going but you know you'll get there with your inner compass. And if there are hurdles in your way, positivity will help you either jump over them or go around them – or, better yet, embrace them, not as your adversaries but as your allies. They are what make you stronger and help you realize that there's absolutely nothing you can't do, as Sabine indicates. No matter what your circumstances, you CAN survive and thrive!

IMPORTANT MESSAGE:

You may be asking how one can survive and thrive in a situation where the outcome may include death. How can you talk about surviving and thriving when you know the "Angel of Death" may be visiting?

Remember that your life situation is not who you are. When you have inner peace, knowing all is as it should be, you can graciously accept your circumstances, no matter how dire they are, and live every precious moment as if it were your last. Then you will have lived your life to its fullest. You will have survived and thrived!

EXERCISE

When you feel yourself getting depressed or down because of your circumstances, visualize a special place you can go that brings you peace, joy and comfort. Imagine all the sensations of this place...the feelings of safety...of comfort...of joy. Listen to the sounds...notice the smells...taste and touch whatever you wish to touch. Allow yourself to experience everything about this place, the peace and joy and tranquility and comfort and safety. Let these feelings intensify and become a part of you, imprinted on your heart and mind, taken deep within you.

Know how you feel when you go to this special place; and whenever you focus your mind on this place, the feelings return immediately. So when you experience anxiety or depression or doubt or fear, know that you can return to this special place where you are safe, at peace, and full of joy. And when possible, as you are in your special place in your mind, bring the feelings with you, into your outer reality, feeling the same joy and peace and comfort and safety in your outer surroundings, with the people around you, during your activities.

And when you do this, ask yourself: is your perception of things around you different as you emanate this special place outward?

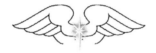

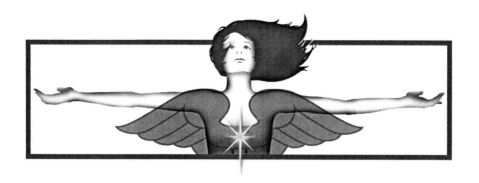

Shaping the Future:
Getting a New Lease on Life

*"Take one day at a time and enjoy each precious moment....
Live your life to the fullest, as there is no time to waste!"*

I was watching *North and South* the other night, a saga about the Civil War, and as it ended, I started getting very upset and began crying. I had begun to think of the day I had my stroke and I was overwhelmed with emotion. It was like I had just had the stroke and was going through the grieving stage. But why now, after almost two years after that fateful day? Why was I so distressed now since I was 90% recovered and I could finally see the light at the end of the tunnel? And why did this happen as I was watching the end of *North and South*, when the two families who had been on opposing sides reunited and were preparing to rebuild all they had lost during the war?

I first thought back to when I had the stroke to see what my feelings were then and I realized that I never felt anything...as if I had been "numb" to the whole situation, or as my mom put it, I was "blasé" about the whole thing. I determined that I was just in denial of what was happening to me, which is a necessary stage you go through when facing a life-changing challenge. My mom even told me that, at the hospital, I asked her, "Why is this happening?" but I don't remember saying that, as I must have been in and out of consciousness.

And now, all of a sudden, I began to feel the despair I should have felt at the beginning, after the denial. And what was the trigger that caused me to come to this place of utter despondency, when things were actually going well? And why as I was watching *North and South*? I mulled over it for a while because the "ah-ha" didn't come as quickly as usual. This time, I had to piece it together. And I concluded that this was because I was coming from a place of anxiety and fear of not being able to figure it out, instead of surrendering and letting Spirit speak through me. I realized I was at another level of healing, purging remnants of the surfacing anxieties that had plagued me for so long. It takes time to undo thoughts and behaviors that are deeply rooted in your psyche, and apparently I still had some pesky inner critters trying to seduce me into the darkness, keeping me from seeing with clarity. It didn't take long, though, to see what was going on. In order to clear my mind so the truth could shine through, I went and grabbed something to eat, letting my mind wander until it hit upon the answer.

I concluded that my despondency was a delayed response to my situation. Although I had accepted my circumstance for what it was, I hadn't grieved over it. Okay, maybe I do things backwards (my son has told me I'm crazy!), but everybody has their own way of dealing with things. I also learned that I wasn't alone in what was happening to me. I blasted a message of my predicament to all the stroke association pages on Facebook I was following, to see if others had gone through the same thing, and the answer I received from many was a resounding, "Yes, it's a normal part of the process, but we do it in our own way." I got many stories of how others had dealt with their emotions throughout their recovery.

So there it was. My grieving at this late stage of the game was necessary for me to progress further along the road to recovery. You must always allow yourself to feel all the emotions you go through during your recovery. You should never hold them in, or they will fester and settle in your body and cause further illness. You should release all emotions in whatever way you can that's safe and not detrimental to yourself or to others.

And the reason why *North and South* triggered the emotions was this. The movie was about two factions at war with each other, kind of like the inner imbalance I struggled with between the masculine and feminine principles. At the end of the movie, signifying the end of the war, the two factions reunite. That is, the two families who were on opposing sides during the war. The family from the north helps the family from the south rebuild their homestead, which they have lost. And wasn't that what my stroke was all about – my feminine side helping to rebuild my masculine side, which had been put out of commission, both psychologically and physically, and thus creating unity between the two? Just like the two families were reuniting and rebuilding their lives after the war, I too was establishing the inner balance I so desired after my own battle and, thus, reshaping my future with a new lease on life.

Read now how Tina viewed her life after being diagnosed with cancer that metastasized.

"To say that my February 2010 breast cancer diagnosis threw me for a loop would be a decided understatement. I couldn't remember a time when I felt as good. I was happy, working hard, and having fun. As I remember it, the 4x3 centimeter lump appeared seemingly overnight. I had just been to my OB/GYN to have my IUD replaced three weeks prior. I had a breast exam at the time. There was nothing there. I assumed at first it was a blocked duct or cyst and expected it to start to hurt or feel hot.

When it didn't, I made an appointment and was referred for a mammogram – at age 43, my first. I had to wait three days but wasn't particularly worried because I expected I would be told what my OB/GYN had suggested, that I was experiencing 'fibrocystic breast change'.

"*The radiologist stood and started talking as we closed the distance between us. 'Hi. You have a tumor and we need to get it out as soon as possible. There is a surgeon upstairs who has agreed to meet with you at 3:00 today. Can you be there?'*

"'*I'm sorry. What?'*

"'*Is someone here with you today?'*

"'*No!'*

"*He offered me his hand, but not a seat.*

"*Everyone agrees: there was no reason for my cancer. No family history. I gave birth twice. I breastfed my children. No previous mammograms or chest x-rays. I rarely drank alcohol, walked three miles at least four times a week, and was within an acceptable weight range. I spent a considerable amount of time wondering not so much 'how' but 'why.' What was I supposed to learn from the experience?*

"*I remember everyone telling me (as if I were considering the alternative), 'You have so much to live for. Do it for your boys.' Three months into treatment, I realized that living for someone else isn't a good enough reason to poison and torture your body the way mine was being poisoned and tortured. You have to do it for yourself.*

"I had a lumpectomy, a mastectomy, six rounds of chemo (Carboplatin and Taxotere), Herceptin infusions every three weeks for a year, five weeks of radiation, and two reconstructive surgeries before I was diagnosed with brain metastasis on Valentine's Day 2012. Clearly, whatever I was supposed to learn 1) hadn't been learned and 2) was important. I am still in treatment today and still wondering what it is.

"What most people find difficult to understand is that I wouldn't change a thing about my life. Every person, event, and decision has brought me to who I am today – and I like who I am. Someone once told me I had a charmed life, which, at face value, is far from true. I realized it wasn't that I had a charmed life, but that I looked at my circumstances as just that – circumstances. They were only bad or good if I ascribed one meaning or the other to them. As such, I began ascribing good meaning, even to the unpleasant ones. After all, they have all made me a wiser and more empathic person.

"When we see people running or biking, my boyfriend often comments, 'Everyone wants to live forever. Why is everyone afraid to die?' I realized that, while I have no desire to leave the people I love, I am not afraid of death. Sort of like a fear of falling is often called a fear of heights – I don't think people fear death – I think people fear the manner in which they will ultimately die. No one wants a painful, blood-soaked, fear-filled death – who would? Over the past few years, people have extolled my bravery and courage. Bravery and courage? What is it about me doing the only thing I know how to do (i.e., live) that is so brave or courageous?

"When I think about dying, what breaks my heart is the inevitable sadness my loved ones will experience. I don't

like the idea of being the cause of sadness. I would like to be remembered for the times I made people laugh. I have promised my boys, 18 and 16 now, that whenever they need me, I will be there. That they know me well enough to know exactly what I would say. That even if I died tomorrow, we are so lucky to have known each other so well and for so long.

"Despite the metastasis, I am not convinced cancer will kill me. I believe I am too busy living for death to sneak in. I have a theory that you can't die in the present moment – that if the present moment is taken up by life, there is no room for death. Maybe this is how I get out of bed in the morning and get down to the business of living each day."

As I was reading Tina's story when she first sent it to me, it brought to light something that was still somewhat of a concern to me. A part of me still questioned whether I would fully recover, even though I knew deep down that I would. The past few weeks had made me think otherwise. My body was in rebellion, it seemed. My right side was stiff and unyielding, and my walking was stilted and unsteady. In rehab, I found myself scared to do some of the exercises the therapists were asking me to do, even though I knew they were pushing me harder so that I COULD recover. The only way I was going to make progress was to work harder, to push myself, not like I used to out of force, but out of determination and perseverance, a wanting to get better. I had gone through this before, but not with the same magnitude of emotion behind the resistance. Was I in denial again? Was I grieving what I had lost, my old life when I could dance and move so freely? How could I pull myself out of the funk I had fallen into?

Then I thought about what I said at the end of the last chapter "You Can Survive and Thrive":

"Remember that your life situation is not who you are. When you have inner peace, knowing all is as it should be, you can graciously accept your circumstances, no matter how dire they are, and live every precious moment as if it were your last!"

Isn't that what Tina meant when she said, "If the present moment is taken up by life – there is no room for death"? You know the saying, "Yesterday is history, tomorrow is a mystery, but today is a gift; that's why it's called the 'present.'"

As Tom Hanks said in the movie *Forest Gump*, "Life is like a box of chocolates; you never know what you're going to get." This is so true! We are presented with opportunities from one minute to the next throughout our lives, good and bad. When the opportunity comes in the form of a life-altering experience such as illness, our choices of how to handle it will either propel us forward on a journey of inner peace or make us sink in the quicksand of despair. Look at the trauma as a gift of the soul and see how it can transform you into a different person, a better person. Take one day at a time and enjoy each precious moment. Appreciate the little things in life. Cherish yourself and your loved ones. Be adventurous and embrace new challenges with fervor. Take the road less travelled. Seek out what gives meaning to your life and go after it passionately. Live your life to the fullest, as there is no time to waste!

EXERCISE

In your journal or notebook, write down the things that give you a new lease on life. What things do you want to do that give you purpose in life, that you are passionate about? Put them in order of priority and see how you can fulfill your dreams by pursuing them one at a time.

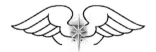

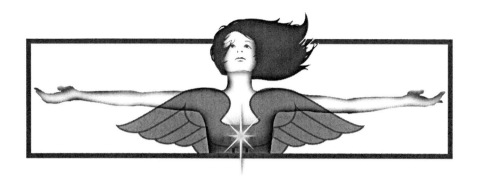

Miracles Do Happen

"When you believe in yourself and your connection to Spirit and its power, you open yourself up to new possibilities. Miracles are real! They do happen!"

Y ou're probably tired of hearing me say this, but each time I've needed to deal with something, the chapter I began to write was based on that issue or emotion. In the case of this chapter, it wasn't really some issue or underlying emotion I had to work on, such as believing in myself or surrendering or limiting beliefs or most of the themes in the other chapters. It was actually what happened to me two days before I began this chapter; and of course, just as with the other chapters, I felt compelled to write about it! A miracle happened!

A few days before I began, I was written up on a stroke organization's website. They posted my story of why I had a stroke. Of course, I actually wrote it, but they edited it to fit their needs and placed it on their website. You already know my story has both a physical component to it (the hole in my heart that allowed a blood clot to pass through to my brain) and a spiritual element (finding inner harmony by shifting from an ego-based masculine mindset to one that is more feminine and heart-centered). Well, Mom and I were watching

TV, as is typical just before going to bed, and I began thinking about my book launch and the funding campaign and all I had to do for both. I had only one month before kicking off my funding campaign and only four months before the book launch...not really a lot of time considering what each entailed.

Would I really have the time to run a successful campaign and launch within the timeframe? That question had been nagging at me for some time. Then Spirit hit me on the head, gently of course. Why did I feel like I had to launch my book on June 10, 2013? Granted, that was the two-year anniversary of my stroke, and it was a special day for me, but if I pushed myself too hard to get there, wasn't I operating once again out of that old masculine-driven forcefulness? And who knows! I could have ended up having another stroke or a heart attack or some other stress-related illness. Then what? I wouldn't get there. There would be no book launch.

I shared my concerns with my mom and she said exactly what I was thinking. "Erica," she said, "you are acting just as you did before your stroke. Push, push, push. You're working yourself into frenzy, and for what? A date?" She was absolutely right. I was still in that old excessively driven mindset. I used to work 80 hours a week before I had my stroke. It takes time to let go of old behaviors and replace them with new ones. I had been reminded of this several times as I wrote each of the chapters of this book.

Then the miracle happened! I remembered the first sentence of the last paragraph of my story that was published on the stroke association's website. "As she became whole on a psychological level, physically she began to recover the right side of her body." This triggered my decision to postpone my book launch until Thanksgiving time. This was actually my original plan, but because I was completing writing my book so quickly, I wanted to push up the launch date. Push, push, push! The decision to push out my launch date was another psychological shift from the masculine to the feminine, where

I was finding that inner balance I had been seeking. And because of this, I knew my body would follow. My right side would become completely normal again, manifesting an outer harmony with the left feminine side that reflected the evolving inner harmony.

The next day, I went outside to exercise. Since I was finally over the flu and feeling pretty good, I had started jogging around the block once each day. But this day, I decided to go two rounds (1 1/3 miles), one jogging, one walking. This was a milestone for me, as I hadn't done it since before my stroke. Yes, I did the 5K/3 1/2 mile walk/run just two months before in December, but I had the owner of the rehab center with me encouraging me all the way. And since I was with the rehab therapists and was only one of three patients participating in the run, it was very motivating. But I did this walk all by myself, with self-support only. My goal was to go around five times (three miles) like I used to do, and I knew I could do it. My body was really feeling like it was going to return to normal. Actually, because of all the exercise I was doing alongside my rehab, I would probably be even better than before. And so the miracle continued.

Miracles can happen, and they don't have to be something huge. Look for miracles in the smallest of things. "Be open for miracles and listen to the first nudge – don't wait for the big ones! Trust that inner voice and the messages you get...!" These are the word of wisdom of Cherry-Lee, whose near-death experience during childbirth became her miracle.

"I had a miserable pregnancy with my first daughter. I slept poorly and threw up excessively every day for the 34 weeks of my pregnancy. I was a first grade teacher at the time and it was incredibly challenging to work full-time and manage a classroom of students with repeated trips to the children's bathroom to vomit. I felt ill throughout the entire pregnancy and had this niggling sense that something was wrong. At around the seven-

month mark, I had a regular check-up. I had been feeling particularly horrible and found out I had PIH (Pregnancy-Induced Hypertension) or Pre-Eclampsia, a life-threatening condition. I was put on IMMEDIATE bed rest. No more teaching elementary school for the year. I didn't even have a chance to say goodbye to my students.

"*During that time, my doctor reassured us that I would know what was needed, and to trust my intuition and my husband's. She felt I was in good hands because my husband was also a doctor – a family doctor.*

"*In spite of her reassurances, my doctor became hyper-vigilant. She sent me to a Perinatologist in Tacoma, Washington, to make sure my baby was okay. He was also concerned and explained it was a waiting game. The longer the baby stayed inside me, the more likely she would come out without issue. And yet, the longer she stayed inside me, the sicker I would get. The goal was to find the optimal time for the two of us, as it was potentially fatal for me. If she came out early, she might have undeveloped lungs and more. He measured and she was quite small for her gestational age. He gave me steroids to help her develop. I underwent repeated tests to monitor my condition.*

"*After a couple weeks of extensive doctors' visits and testing, I was at home one day and not feeling well. I had a friend from the school stop by and visit me. She expressed concern that I shouldn't be left alone, so she stayed until my husband got home. I felt her love and compassion, and honestly it scared me. The next morning I told my husband I didn't want him to go to work. He said, 'That makes it easy. If you don't want me away from you, I don't want you out of the hospital.' We called the doctor, packed my things and he drove me to* the hospital. He left me there for the day while he intuitively made preparations to be off of work for a while. On my own, I signed my living will with the help of another dear teacher friend. My fear was escalating as we took these practical steps.

"Wayne didn't get back to me until 10:00 pm, at which point I was starving and really ill. I ate some salad he had brought me and then threw it all up. I didn't even really try to sleep, and I was feeling sicker by the minute. Wayne rubbed and rubbed my feet, and I could hardly feel his hands. As the night went on, I realized I couldn't pee. I asked for a catheter because the pressure was so intense. The nurse didn't agree that I needed one and argued with me. Finally, she inserted one and nothing happened. I didn't understand why. It was at this point that she and Wayne began to get stressed because I was in renal (kidney) failure.

"The next thing that happened was I felt this gush. I felt such relief. I thought my water had broken and I mentioned this to Wayne, who immediately called the nurse. It turned out that my placenta had erupted and I was lying in a pool of blood. Within minutes they moved me to an operating room and began surgery. I later learned my doctor had been asked to leave another surgery to come take care of me. She left them in good hands, I was reassured.

"My doctor had to perform a vertical C-section because my blood wasn't clotting properly. Non-clotting blood is called DIC and is something that happens in end-stage AIDS patients with septic shock and other extreme cases. They knew that delivering the baby would LIKELY begin my healing process – if I made it.

151

"They took the baby out roughly and sewed me up quickly, hoping my blood would begin to clot and my kidneys would kick back in.

"The baby, my eldest daughter Avalon, came out at 4 lbs 2 oz and with a very low APGAR score. On a scale of 1 to 10, she scored a 2. She had one point for being blue instead of grey and one point for an irregular heartbeat. She was taken to the special care nursery. My husband looked at my doctor, asking her what to do. She said, 'Go with the baby – we've done all we can for your wife. It's a waiting game now.'

"So, he went and was present while Avalon was cared for by a nurse in the special care unit. The nurse, Elly, was a Healing Touch Certified Practitioner and Shaman, working in Saint Peter's hospital. She gave Avalon a bath, did a healing session and massaged her with lavender oil. Avalon's APGAR score went from that initial 2 to an 8 within 10 minutes. The rising score was truly a miracle to us, as Avalon had stopped growing in utero.

"Recovering from surgery, I came to but was in and out of consciousness. I was put on anti-seizure medication and was still very swollen from the kidney failure. The nurses brought Avalon to me later that day. My vision was so messed up that I saw her in triplicate. I had many visiting friends and specialists. I couldn't see who to look at when they spoke, as everyone came in multiples. They placed Avalon on my belly and I couldn't even feel her. I had no sensation in my fingers – or any part of me – because of the fluid build-up.

"I continued drifting in and out of consciousness for hours. I heard later of the healer who had helped Avalon. I asked for her to come to me. She did. Somewhere in there, I went through a tunnel of rainbow-

colored light. It was like I was on my hospital bed but rainbow streamers were flowing by. I went to a place that was very light and my granny was there (who had passed away when I was three). I remember feeling Granny's presence again and knowing everything would be okay.

"After Elly worked on me, I began to heal. My kidneys kicked back in and my wound began to heal. The blood properly clotted, and I started my slow road to recovery. My doctor said that since I was beginning to rebuild, she didn't want to give me a transfusion. It still took a LONG time to build my blood back up. It was three weeks before I could even walk and carry my tiny baby because my balance, strength and sense of being upright were just OFF! I truly think it was a miracle that this nurse/healer was there. I felt that Granny knew we would be okay, and miraculously we were!"

Miracles happen when one believes, when one has faith in the power of the Universe, in the presence of Spirit (God, our co-creator). Miracles happen every day. We just have to open our eyes to see them. One that often happens to me is what I call "parking lot karma." Most every time I pull into a parking lot and look for a parking spot, undoubtedly no matter how full the parking lot is, there's one close to the entrance of where I need to go, or someone is pulling out just as I am pulling up. (I wish I could transfer this karma to my finances! Maybe one day!)

A miracle can seem like an impossibility, like when a metastasized tumor becomes benign or when someone blind can suddenly see. But miracles are founded in faith, the belief that a Higher Power is at work. The mother of Joel Osteen, the widely acclaimed senior pastor at Lakewood Church in Houston, Texas, was diagnosed with liver cancer in 1981 and told she had only a few weeks to live. But through a strong faith, the power of prayer and support, and visualizing herself as well, she is alive and healthy today. When you believe in yourself and your connection to Spirit and its power, you open yourself up to new possibilities. "If our hearts and minds are open and loving, we will find our right path and our true self. There will be signs illuminating and confirming the way."[27]

Miracles are real! They do happen!

EXERCISE

In your journal or notebook, think back through your life and write down all the times when a miracle happened, big or small. You may be amazed at all the times you may have passed up as "coincidence" or "happenstance" that were actually miracles happening in your life.

~ OR ~

Make a "Miracle jar" much like the Gratitude jar in the "Gratitude and Attitude" chapter. Each time a miracle happens in your life, write it down and place it in the jar. After a period of time, take them all out and see how many have occurred during that time.

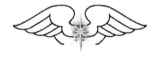

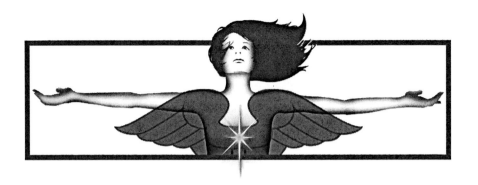

The Caregiver's
Side of the Story

> *"The caregiver goes through his or her own recovery by accepting the current situation and moving forward with a new story.... What are the small moments that can bring us joy and happiness in the new life set before us? This is what we should shoot for!"*

This book has been primarily from the survivor's viewpoint, but I would like to use this chapter to present the caregiver's perspective of dealing with life-altering experiences, since the caregivers are also deeply affected by the challenges of their charges. In some cases, they are more traumatized by the circumstances than the patient, as was my mom.

Please note that other than my mom's story, these stories are not from the caregivers of those who have shared their stories in this book. Instead, they are stories from other caregivers who have shared their own tales of survival in dealing with the trauma of their charges.

This chapter is much longer than any of the other chapters in this book, because it comprises multiple stories instead of just one. They are all special stories, as are all the survivor stories, and show the different perspectives of being a caregiver. The last story is an endearing tale about a woman who takes care of her disabled dog and how it transforms her life, and how she uses her experience to help others with disabled dogs. Dogs are like children, in the eyes of many!

My Mom's Story

"I wish to share my mom's story, not from her eyes but from mine. The reason is that Mom was much more traumatized by my stroke than I was and she chose not to relive it again by writing about it. I hope you will understand why, as I tell you her story.

"Mom has been a caregiver since she was eight years old when her own mom had a stroke at 36 years old. Being the oldest girl of an Italian peasant family of four children, my mom had to take on the domestic chores of an adult, thus never being able to just be a child. She rarely got to play, since she was always too busy accommodating the needs of the family.

"Her caregiving continued into her adult life when my father was diagnosed with emphysema, which took his life when he was 50 years old. For the last eight years of his life, from the time of his diagnosis to the time of his death in 1982, Mom worked three jobs, raised two children (my brother and me), got her Ph.D. (she has four degrees) and took care of my father. And because my mom is a saint at heart, she would also take in anyone who had serious personal issues and needed support. Through the years, our home was like a shelter for strays. All of this culminated in my having a stroke. Because I couldn't take care of myself, at least in the beginning, I moved in with my mom, while my younger

son who lived with me before the stroke moved in with his father.

"When I first had my stroke, my mother was devastated when the ER doctor said I could die. She had already been through so much hardship in her life, and to think that she now might lose a child was too much to handle. Fortunately, I survived; however, the road to my recovery was a very hard journey for Mom. Think about it! She was 75 years old when I had my stroke, a time when she should have been retired from work, yet she still had to work to make ends meet. She was a university professor, teaching three classes, grading umpteen papers, attending conferences, presenting papers, and sitting on various university committees...all the things required of a university professor. AND she was taking care of me.

"In the beginning, I needed a lot of care, and needless to say, it was very hard for Mom to keep up with all she had to do between her job and being my caregiver. Her health suffered, as did her spirit. She has always been my rock, but this period of time chipped away at her undying strength and zest. As I recovered, things did become easier as I became more self-sufficient. When I had the strength and energy, I would do what I could around the house to offload some of the chores from Mom.

"As time went on, life did become more and more normal; however, it didn't return to what it was before. It actually became better because we both had a transformation of self. It was an extremely difficult journey, but we both made it through. My mom and I have a very special relationship, our lives running parallel. Mom had spent much of her life on a very

profound spiritual quest, as had I on a different level, and our journeys had come to the end of the road together.

"We are now at the beginning of our new lives, just waiting to see what magic will come forth."

Lynn's Story

"The chiming of the telephone ring provided no clue about how our life was about to be turned upside down. The frosty December morning in 2007, much like any other in Maryland, now stands out poignantly in our memories. Dad's doctor was calling to tell him to check into the hospital right away – his recent blood work warranted further testing that could not wait. Having had a heart attack that required five-bypass surgery almost 19 years earlier, he followed his doctors' instructions to the letter. He wanted to live! Just as calmly as Dad had informed Mom that he needed to get to the hospital immediately, years before, she was ready to go one more time. She knew to ask questions later.

"A few days of testing brought devastating news: Dad had multiple myeloma, a blood cancer. Incurable. Uncommon. Cancer! Despite our initial shock, it mobilized us to learn whatever we could about this disease: What was it? What treatments worked? Side effects? Risks? Prognosis? Dad's oncologist could not answer the obvious question: How long would Dad remain with us? His age was a factor working against him. Dad was 81.

"Mom, my brother, my sister and I, as well as our spouses, became a well-oiled caregiving machine, a team focused solely on taking care of Dad. All of us

*applied our particular talents and skills to helping him –
be it researching medications, treatments or what to
expect from the disease, driving him to dialysis three
times a week, shopping for groceries and refilling his
meds, finding comfortable clothes, cooking nutritious
meals that he would actually tolerate and eat, or looking
for services and support. It was the least we could do for
our beloved father. He was a loving, down-to-Earth,
humble man who could find a way to make you smile, to
bring out the greatness in us even when we could not
see it ourselves.*

*"I am sure that in the back of our minds, all of us
wondered how long Dad would be able to fight this
cancer. We focused on doing what we could to make his
existence a meaningful one every day. Whether it was
through conversation or simply sitting with him, we
wanted him to know beyond the shadow of a doubt that
he was loved more than he could imagine. And he was. I
think he knew. We sometimes felt the fear of losing our
sweet father; while at other times, we were at peace and
accepting of the finality of life. As adult children, we had
never discussed our parents' mortality. The close call
that presented itself 19 years earlier served more as a
wake-up call to make changes for the good than as an
intimidating experience. Dad, especially, saw it as a
second chance at life. He was not finished just yet.*

*"I told my sister one night that, while I hoped and
prayed daily for Dad, when I thought about his future, I
saw black. In my mind, no image or place or action
appeared. Only black. I took this as a sign that our dear
father would not be with us very long. I had no idea how
long, just not long. What I found very strange, and yet
totally comfortable at the same time, was that I felt a
sense of tranquility and acceptance. A given, like*

reading a passage of what is to come. I know my faith is the main factor that allowed me to cope with this tremendous loss. A loss that words cannot begin to express. A loss that no other human understands until he or she has experienced it. I also know the profound love and amazing support from our family and friends were an important part of the healing process that continues today.

"I missed my Dad's passing. My sister told me she had a feeling he may not last much longer, about one or two weeks before he left this world. I believed he would be around a little longer because his condition was unstable and seemed to dispense false alarms at random. I live in Austin, Texas and planned to fly to Maryland when it became evident that his time had come. I waited a little too long, but managed to speak to him a couple hours before he died. I was told that his last words were spoken to me. I was with him in spirit and he knows I love him still.

"Reflecting on Dad's final moments, I told my sister that I could not imagine what it was like to see him go. I have a mental picture of my sister and brother, their spouses and our mother at his bedside, waiting. My sister saw it differently: I had been spared.

"Never in a million years did I envision my husband becoming disabled as Dad's condition was deteriorating, having to give up his meaningful career as a scientist, and me becoming a caregiver once again. I had missed Dad's departure, which came almost four months after his diagnosis, but perhaps I will get my turn in time. I do believe firmly in Destiny, that a path is set for us to follow by our Divine Savior and that His will encourages us to do good. Along with the challenges that He sends

us, He sends the strength to deal with them, I have read. This gives me courage and hope. It is my faith that enables me to endure and to rise above hardship. I know I don't have to understand how this works. It suffices that I know it does!

"As much as our Lord plans for us, however, He also says He helps those who help themselves. To that end, I approach family caregiving as a project: I research and learn about my husband's condition (CRPS – Complex Regional Pain Syndrome); I organize his medical records, medications, notes, insurance papers, Will, Advance Directives, Power of Attorney (medical and durable), and any other documents; I prepare nutritious meals; I find medical services that come to our home in order to avoid the painful ride in a car to the doctor's office, etc. My husband and I are also a great team: we work together to find solutions regarding his care; we are open-minded and creative when looking for ways to accommodate his limited mobility and very painful existence; we persevere until a suitable option is found; we look for the good in every situation, no matter how bad something seems to be. We also keep humor, a positive attitude, patience, love and respect for one another in the forefront. This doesn't mean we don't have bad days; we do. But we don't let them stop us or defeat us. We have a choice of outlook in every situation: we can sink or swim. We choose to swim!

"Some of the biggest challenges we have faced with Dad and with my husband have been finding ways to keep them comfortable through their pain and serving meals they enjoyed. Pain patches or medications took away the edge of the pain. What has worked best with my husband has been distraction. He feels his pain 24/7. His only respite is sleep, which is short and light. As for

161

food, my father used to say it tasted like cardboard, probably due to the chemotherapy. My husband's faulty nervous system sends the 'wrong' signals throughout the body, changing the flavor or aroma of many foods to unpalatable ones. So what do you feed someone who finds food disgusting? In our case, small amounts of foods that are fresh, colorful, and not too aromatic or spicy worked best. And no nagging to clean your plate!

"I think the biggest challenge of all has been seeing our loved ones suffer day in and day out. Knowing they will continue to face their condition without a reasonable chance of improvement, and most likely continued deterioration, is difficult to live with for both patient and caregiver. Eroding independence to perform even the simple tasks can (erroneously) feel like incompetence and an imposition on family and friends. It can happen ever so gradually, like the straw that broke the camel's back, that it takes us by surprise. It can feel like the patient is as helpless as a child, leaving your loved one feeling vulnerable and embarrassed. This presents another challenge: reassuring the patient that none of the lost abilities defines the person. Just because my husband can no longer cut his meat due to pain and stiffness in his hands, or finds a spoon easier to use, it does not make him any less of an adult. While I know I am not responsible for their physical demise or for their cure, seeing my father or my husband suffer so much, physically or emotionally, has been overwhelming sometimes. I prayed then and pray now for relief and for strength for my husband to get past the misery.

"As our caregiving journey continues (and it is a journey on which the entire family embarked five years ago), my husband strives to remain as self-sufficient as possible. He knows, however, that the time will come when he

will need help or I will have to perform certain tasks for him. We are prepared for that, but continue to give him opportunities to do as much as he can on his own. He still walks on crutches instead of being in a wheelchair. He eats his food with a spoon, cut into pieces, not too hot or spicy. He drinks water from a tall covered thermal bottle with a loop for easier handling. He has what he needs within reach, including little treats to enjoy. He has an iPad to communicate with the world and stay in touch with family and friends; to keep his mind sharp with research, news, paying bills online, reading books or doing mental calisthenics; and to find amusing diversions like movies or jokes. He is surrounded by greeting cards wishing him well and reminding him that he is not alone or forgotten. We talk about everything, including how we are feeling and our vision for the near future. We haven't talked much about life in the far future, other than that we would love to live in France or England! I have promised him that on his last day on Earth, I will bring him a given-up-due-to-meds pint of Stout or a glass of Glenfiddich if he so desires!

"My caregiving journey also includes being a long-distance caregiver for my mother, which started when Dad passed away. Both roles evolve as needs arise or change. I see myself continuing to look for ways to make life pleasant and meaningful for both my husband and my mother. I also find it immensely rewarding to share information and resources with other family caregivers. I know that becoming a family caregiver is usually an unplanned decision, which results from compassion and the desire to help. Unfortunately, we begin this chapter with little or no training or concept of what the job entails. To address that, I created a website that provides useful links to information, resources and support for family caregivers: CaregivingCafe.com. My

goal is to help family caregivers better manage their own caregiving journey, and to encourage them to practice self-care. After all, a strong and effective caregiver is a healthy and informed caregiver!"

Suzanne's Story

"Like every human being on this planet, life has always had its ups and downs. My parents separated while I was in high school and I was the oldest of seven. While high school should be carefree and fun, my years were full of conflict and responsibility. As I look back, once I got married the years had a sense of fun and adventure during my twenties. I later loved being a mom to my children, Steven and Kristin, and wife to David. The years were busy with work I loved, going back to college and getting my BA and MA. Life was full, lots of love and laughter.

"On October 28, 2001, my world changed dramatically. David was a Boy Scout leader and on this beautiful fall day, he and my son headed out for a 50-mile bike ride. David left that morning after telling me it would be a piece of cake. I had a stew and an apple crisp brewing for their return and we would plan our Halloween festivities carving pumpkins and baking pumpkin seeds when they returned. I received a phone call in the afternoon from one of the scout moms that changed our lives forever. David had a heart attack. She didn't know the details or chose not to tell me at the time.

"When I arrived at the hospital, my son was sitting in the waiting room with a chaplain. At that moment, I knew it was not going to be good news. David was unconscious after cardiac arrest. They did not believe he would make it through the night. Family gathered

around. I slept on the couch in the waiting room while his youngest brother slept in the room with him, not wanting him to be alone if he passed on.

"Three days later, to the doctors' and nurses' shock, David came out of the coma. Unfortunately, after tests, he was brain-injured and would be disabled the rest of his life. The lack of oxygen to the brain caused permanent damage to his motor skill and short-term memory faculties. My beautiful 48-year-old genius husband was changed forever. The next six months were spent in many hospitals and nursing home facilities, learning to navigate a new life full of specialists, physical and occupational therapies, speech therapy and nurses, as well as trying to take care of my home and children.

"On April 26, 2002, on his birthday, David came home. Our home would turn into a place of wheelchairs, handrails and other equipment. For the next five years, I became David's caregiver. As difficult a journey as it was, I was thankful that he was still with us. I took on my new role at first full of promise and high hopes that he would be well again, and did everything I could with conventional and alternative healing to assist him. Although the doctors had said there was little hope for any change, I wanted to prove them wrong.

"For the first two years, David did make some improvement and he too had hope. About four years in, he was very weary, frustrated and tired of the battle. It was clear to us that his soul had made a decision: he wanted to leave soon. Our daughter begged him not to give up. We all seemed to make a collective agreement that we would get our son through high school the next year. In the back of my mind, I felt I would then convince

him to get our daughter through high school, but that would be a LONG four more years and David had already made up his mind: he'd had enough of the struggle.

"On our son's graduation, David was in an amazingly happy mood. We thought he was just really proud of our son. And then it dawned on me. He had kept our agreement. He could now leave when he was ready. Less than two months later, David passed away at the age of 53 for his own new beginning without the struggle of a body that could no longer function. Everyone loved David. He was an amazing husband, dad, engineer, world traveler, Boy Scout leader, diplomat, friend, brother, son and a 'beloved' gift to the world, as his name was so aptly chosen. His beautiful smile, his twinkling eyes and his kindly smile that our son wrote of him in a dedication poem will never be forgotten, for all who met and knew him.

"During the time of David's disability in 2005, my youngest brother, NJ, also became disabled. He fell in the shower at his home and is now a quadriplegic and lives in a nursing home. NJ is an amazing soul. We call him an earth angel. Friends from his school days come to see him. At my Dad's funeral, I said to a couple friends how grateful I was to them for spending time with him. They told me it is an honor to be with him; he is an inspiration to them and that is why they go. I truly believe he is here to show us through his struggles, so we can keep a spirit of love, joy and kindness.

"Through these major challenges, and then the illness and passing of my dad, and now my mother who is at Stage 4 with cancer, I sometimes wonder if I have been given more challenges than most. What is the purpose of

all these challenges? I felt that a sense of purpose did prevail through my experience with my husband. I learned a level of patience and unconditional love that was deeper than I had thought possible. My sense of humor got me through many difficult days. The bottom line is that everything we experience is either love or fear and what we choose. These experiences have helped me choose love more than fear. Every day, every moment, is this choice.

"I found I had a purpose: to support others, and to re-create their lives through my work as a life coach. During troubles, we often lose the passion, purpose and playfulness of our lives. This was my purpose, to support others with new beginnings, often after difficult and challenging times. The Universe had given me these opportunities to walk the talk of the spiritual path, and then to be able to support others to do the same.

"I also learned we must work through and clear the grief that gets stored in our bodies, often leading to health challenges and illness. We often believe we have worked through the grief, and then when a new challenge hits us, we boomerang back to unresolved issues that have not been fully cleared. For me, this came when my golden retriever passed away. My wonderful dog gave my children and me an opportunity again to heal on a deeper level.

"It is a time for new beginnings. I am ready to embark on a new chapter in my life, which will allow me to continue to bring more passion, purpose and playfulness into my own life experience, as well as support others on their journey. And never give up. There is a reason, a purpose, a deeper meaning that is calling from our souls to become more, to be more. The challenges of our lives

cause us to dig deep to find out who we truly are. We are stronger and stronger than we ever could imagine. The ebbs and the flow of life are here to teach us that we are spiritual beings living a human experience. And we are more than we can ever know or imagine."

Erica's Story

"In 2007 my husband Jim Young received a misdiagnosis of ALS/Lou Gehrig's disease. Although we eventually got the correct diagnosis of chronic Lyme disease with overlap ALS symptoms, Jim has struggled to maintain his health and life. His neurological and muscular systems have been hit hard. In 2008 he had to have a tracheotomy and feeding tube inserted. Today, Jim is ventilator-dependent and unable to bear weight and walk. And because Jim cannot talk easily (we currently use a letter board to spell out words), a conversation can take a very long time. Still, we see improvements slowly and believe he can still regain his health.

"Jim and I have thought from the beginning that there must be something good we can take from this. Having this perspective helps a great deal. I also know I have been gifted with resilience beyond the average person. I never knew this until the crisis, but it is true that I tend to view things differently to many people I know. In addition to caring for Jim, I am raising our two children (currently ages seven and four), and I have to call in lots of favors to help in this area – and I work full-time. Logistically, trying to get everything done that needs to get done in a day is difficult.

"I do a variety of everyday tasks for Jim and fortunately have nursing help right now, as well. My main duties

include lifting Jim in order to move him various places, making up his food, working hard to get the precise combination of calories, protein and healthy food and then feeding him through his feeding tube. There are other areas in which I help as well, including being a translator at times, since it can be tricky learning how to read the board quickly. A lot of time is spent running errands and following up on things for Jim's needs, including going to the physician's office, filling out forms, answering questions, organizing logistics with care and trying to stay on top of the medical bills.

"As difficult as this predicament is, there are many things that have helped me cope emotionally with our circumstances so I can remain the most resilient, loving wife and mother I can be, while giving myself the love and nurturing that I need, as well. For instance, one of my sisters helped me set up a caringbridge.com site on the internet to let people know about Jim. I would write daily posts and realized I got a lot out of voicing things. I also depended on the lift from people's notes written on the site. They helped a bunch.

"I branched out to write articles for various venues, my blog Traveling Troubled Times *and my website* Bounce to Resilience. *Wanting to find meaning in the crisis and penning my views that belief, faith, and persistence are important when steering your own future became important. And when I could help someone else through an article I wrote or a conversation I had with them, I would be reminded that there is always good to find in the bad.*

"My big project, of which I am most proud, is the book I wrote on my family's experience, Miracles for Daddy: A Family's Inspirational Fight against a Modern Medical

Goliath. *Other smaller things that help a lot include doing 'normal' things with my children and reminding myself how fortunate I am to have these sweet little people in my life. I also don't do it often enough, but yoga and walking around my neighborhood can be quite helpful. Finally, it must be said that talking with my mom and close friends was and remains vital. Being able to complain, question, consider, and cry with these people has allowed emotions to be released that need to be.*

"Most importantly, I have relied heavily on my faith. I know absolutely without a doubt that God has sent people to tell us things and help us along the way. I know definitely that prayer, both mine and that offered up by friends and family, has gotten us to where we are today. And I believe that if you have faith as small as a mustard seed, you can say to a mountain, 'Move from here to there,' and it will move. Again, this perspective and mindset takes me far. I am still waiting on my mountain to move completely, but I think it has taken baby steps along its track!

"Before his condition, Jim was manager of a group that trained sales people to sell effectively. He was also a trainer in that group. He did go back to work for a year after he had his tracheotomy and was able to breathe on his own for 12-15 hours a day, and walk and talk; however, the role of manager was too difficult and Jim went back to 'individual contributor' as a trainer. And for pleasure, Jim loved to golf and ski when he was healthy. He also loved a good movie, a good restaurant and a good bottle of wine. Now, unfortunately, it is difficult to do any of these things. We try to go out as a family to see kid movies, baseball games, or neighborhood outings, and Jim also watches a lot of TV.

Life is much different to what it was before, but we are still a family and we try to concentrate on the positive interactions we still have with one another.

"Things continue to be an up and down battle. Jim was doing great recently, gaining strength with exercises and physical therapy. He was also seeing improvements with breathing and overall stamina (based on some new treatments we are trying). But then, unfortunately, his lungs collapsed 50% on both sides and after a 2-week hospital stay, he is working again to gain momentum.

"I believe Jim can get well. I know the road is long – it has been hard and it will continue to be difficult – but because I have faith that Jim can be cured, at some point I guess this means I will cease being a caregiver and we will carry on with a new life, very different from before but very blessed nonetheless."

Mark's Story

"My father had a stroke in 1976. I dealt with that from 1976 to 1982, the time of his death. My mom had a stroke in 1995. I dealt with that from 1995 to 2003, the time of her death. Oddly enough, their strokes were quite similar. There was some motor impairment on the left side of their bodies. Higher order cognitive functioning was also impaired (e.g. balancing a checkbook). However, their experiences were very different. My father never came to terms with his stroke and began a slow deterioration culminating in his death in 1982. My mother, on the other hand, was always sure she was getting better. It was a powerful lesson. My mother's attitude dramatically improved her quality of life after the stroke.

"I was 14 years old when my father had his stroke. I'd always been the 'baby of the family' and my father was my best friend. On that day, June 6, 1976, I instantly grew up. My mom had some psychological issues and I knew it was my job to carry all of us through this event. (My siblings were significantly older, 16 and 21 years old, and lived out of state. They had their own issues and while they helped out initially, they had to return to their lives.) When my mom had her stroke in 1995, I had a family of my own and was living in a different state. My sister dealt with the stroke at first. On a visit to my mom, I could see that my sister was really not doing what Mom needed, so I moved her closer to me so I could take over.

"With my dad's stroke, I wasn't able to handle the emotions for many years. I squashed the fear to manage the event. Then, as time passed and I could see he was not going to get back to normal, I became angry. I blamed him for many years. I tried to encourage him, help him get back into things he did before. He chose, though, to stay in a self-pitying mode and even seemed to enjoy being weak – requiring others to do everything for him. It was both frustrating and very hard to understand, as a teenager. It was not until sometime later I understood it was not his fault. Eventually, I came to a point where I saw how hard it must have been for him – a vibrant, strong man in control of his life, suddenly weakened and lost. It must have been dreadful for him. I guess now, the self-pity was just how he responded to a massive, life-changing event since I had to help him with many aspects of life: dressing, bathing, and some basic bodily functions early on when he could not get out of bed.

"My mom and I, on the other hand, had not been close since I was very young. She had so many of her own issues in my youth and throughout her stroke/post-stroke period, so my response to her stroke was fairly clinical; I just dealt with managing the situation. Since she was always eager to get back to what she did before, it was easy to encourage her to do so. By the time I moved her to live near me, she just needed help with financial matters and doctor visits. The early portion of recovery in her case was greatly aided by significant therapy. These types of services were not available when my dad has his stroke. They made an enormous difference, along with my mom's attitude.

"The hardest thing I faced being a caregiver was the tremendous feeling of bewilderment and powerlessness. My best friend, my dad, was gone and this body that looked like him was nothing like him at all. With my mom, it was a struggle to find the time to be there as much as she needed and/or wanted.

"They both evolved to the point where they could take care of basic living activities – bathing, cooking and cleaning. I'd say my dad got to this point about 9 months after the stroke. My mom was there in 90 days – again, therapy helped tremendously. They both needed help with 'thought-related' stuff for the rest of their lives. Managing money, scheduling and organizing their lives were always a challenge.

"Neither fully recovered, so I was involved pretty heavily for the remainder of their lives. It sometimes felt like our roles had reversed: I was raising my parents, but unlike children, they no longer changed. Of course, what I cannot determine from these experiences is how much of this role reversal was simply dealing with aging parents.

My father's stroke experience happened during his late 50s to mid 60s. My mom's happened between her early 70s and early 80s.

"As they are both now gone, I've had some time to process these experiences and I've come to see those who've had a stroke differently. Of course, no one chooses to have a stroke. No one chooses to have their lives turned on end and to face major challenges in tasks and activities that were once taken for granted. I believe these experiences have left me with some empathy for those dealing with stroke or other life-changing struggles."

Becki's Story

"My mother was diagnosed with dementia in 2011. I was shocked that this could happen to my mother, but she claimed she was seeing and hearing things, and when we checked the things she was telling us were happening, there was no evidence that they were true. We then knew she was seeing and hearing things that were not there. One instance was when she thought someone was on her porch with a gun, threatening to kill her. She took her gun and fired through her door, and thinking she had either hit or killed this person, she called the police. They called my husband and me, and when we arrived there was nothing to indicate that any of the above was true.

"Emotionally, I was a basket case, and I felt like I was betraying her by having her taken to mental facilities. But it was so bad that it was the only time I could relax and not worry about her, because I knew she was safe for that time.

"I would try to take her to the store and other places when she would go. I paid bills that she forgot about or just did not pay. I tried to be with her as much as I could, but she was convinced I was trying to kill her, so my support for the most part had to be from the sidelines.

"It took over two years to finally get a guardian assigned. I tried and fought to be her guardian, but she is still convinced I am trying to kill her. When the doctor went to evaluate how she would feel if I became her guardian, she told him, 'If Becki becomes my guardian, I will kill myself,' so she was given a court-appointed guardian. That was one of the most heart-wrenching moments of my life. Fortunately, the person appointed knew my parents, so she had a history with my mom. She allowed me to go to my mom's house and take all family-related things: furniture, pictures, jewelry, etc. My house looks like a memorial to Mom, all the antique furniture, pictures and all kinds of stuff packed into our house.

"The hardest thing I've had to deal with is the fact that the strongest woman I know is never going to be normal again, that she is going to have to be cared for for the rest of her life. I remember her when I was younger. Her parents, my grandparents, were both deaf and I would watch Mom speak to them in sign language. It was awe-inspiring. The family all learned sign language so we could all speak to them.

"That led to her profession as an interpreter, and she did some pretty amazing things. She was the first person to go to the Houston Police Department academy and teach the police some basic sign language. She traveled all over the world interpreting. Some of the people she *interpreted for included the Pope in Rome, and both George Bush Sr. and Jr. She was also a freelance interpreter for years and was later hired at Houston Community College to head their interpreter training program.*

"She also ran Project Independence, which was a program designed for people who had a life-changing accident and could no longer do the job they had before. They taught them to do computer programming and then helped place them in jobs at major companies all over Houston. Kathy Whitmore, the mayor of the city at the time, even declared one day to be named after my mom. And she was on the mayor's, Texas governor's and president's committees for people who are handicapped. She's been retired now for 10 years.

"Before her dementia set in, she used to love traveling and visiting friends and new places. Now she keeps herself busy with activities at the assisted living center where she lives and spends a lot of time reading. Unfortunately, because of her unfounded feelings that I want to kill her, I'm not able to spend much time with her. I only go and visit her about once a month because when I do, it sends her into a tailspin and she becomes even more delusional for several days after.

"I have resigned myself to the fact that this is the best it will ever be, from now on. She has never gotten better and will not ever be better. Things will continue as they have for the last year. I will visit and she will be ugly to me, and although I love her, I know this is not my mom mentally anymore."

Bob's Story

"I came downstairs and entered the living room to talk with my father. I noticed he was trying to get out of the chair using only his left side. I rushed around his chair to see that the right side of his face drooped and his right leg wouldn't move. He kept falling down onto his chair and his tongue was hanging out of his mouth. I thought he was having a grand mal seizure, and later found out he'd had a stroke.

"I was scared, especially for my father, but that didn't stop me from following first aid procedures for what I thought was a seizure. I first tried to keep him calm and asked him if he was okay, but he was unable to communicate. He would slump in his chair, so I tried to get him in an upright position to allow air into his body. I also tried to put an aspirin in his mouth, but he kept flashing around. He was so scared! During this period, I called 911 and waited until the EMTs arrived.

"I was Dad's sole caregiver throughout the rest of his life. Since there's no manual on what to do, I felt like I had no support. I felt like I was alone on a ship being tossed around by a storm at sea. But I spent as much time as I could with him and tried to adjust my life to accommodate his needs. Before his stroke, Dad was self-employed in the financial and sales fields. And for leisure, he enjoyed swimming, hiking, the beach, traveling, bowling, playing pool, darts, cribbage, movies, dogs, singing, baseball, and spending time with me. He had also been an eagle scout, and had a real love for history. Post-stroke, Dad still enjoyed movies, the beach, music and his dog. But because his mobility was limited, his traveling simply became long car rides. And of

course, we continued to spend a lot of quality time together until his passing.

"Eleven years after his stroke, my father was okay to return to work, to a point. For a brief time, I had help from an aid, and for the last year of his life, I had him enrolled in an adult day center, which was a big help while I was at work.

"I had the honor and the privilege to be my father's caregiver from August 8, 1999 to February 17, 2012. He had limited recovery by December 1999, when he transitioned from being in a wheelchair to walking on his own, but by 2008 he slowly started to lose some of what he had gained. He began having to use a walker and other forms of aid. And I didn't know it at the time, but several of his organs were beginning to fail also.

"My life has drastically changed now. My father passed away on February 17, 2012, three days after a triple bypass due to 80% blockage in his heart. I was devastated losing my father, because I was so close to him after being his caregiver. I felt like my right arm was ripped off, and I could only feel my arm (Dad). Now a year later, I'm much better. I've had great support from my family and friends. I have to say my mother, Maura, really was and still is there for me. I'm working out, living life to the fullest, and I know my dad is okay right now. I still miss him, but it's time to move on.

"Since Dad passed away, that door has closed. There are new doors I'll open, like being a father and a husband, using my caring and love for my family. Also, I would like to get involved in charity work to help others, or maybe use my experience to aid future caregivers. I feel caregivers are forgotten, and they go through too much not to be recognized and helped."

Michael's Story

"My wife and I have been caregivers in three instances – for my father-in-law who had dementia, my dad who had leukemia, and my mother who had lung cancer and overcame it but now has pancreatic cancer.

"My father-in-law lived alone since his divorce in 1993, so in 2010 we went and 'rescued' him. We didn't exactly know when he had been diagnosed, and when we saw the extent of his disease, it was just sad and horrible what it was doing to him. However, I found it very fascinating the way his mind would create and distort reality. For example, he created a story that his son, who had been in the Navy until his death from a blood clot in his brain, was in Vietnam and stepped on a grenade and was killed as a war hero.

"We had to do everything: help him into the bath, feed him, manage his meds, take him to doctors, clean, wash clothes, etc. It was much like having a young child, and he got worse as time wore on. We took care of him for eight months, but because my wife and I are also disabled, and he was falling a lot, he finally needed 24-hour professional care, so we moved him to a Veteran's Home where he stayed until his passing.

"My dad, who survived bladder cancer and two triple-bypass surgeries starting in 1998 and then was diagnosed with leukemia in 2006, was simple in that he was happy and kind until the end. His skin blistered in these huge areas, and the skin would come off where his kidneys were failing and the waste came out through the skin. He looked like he had an extraordinary case of radiation burn and poisoning, even though he never had that type of treatment. We would sit with him,

179

prepare meals, run errands, dispose of waste when he became bedridden, apply lotion for radiation burn on his worst areas and comfort him. He was in pretty good shape with the disease until September 2008, and then on December 22 of the same year, he passed away.

"My mother, diagnosed with lung cancer in 2011 and pancreatic cancer this year (2013), is still quite capable of most things. Mostly we have to run errands for her, prepare meals, help with money, clean her house and we pray over her often. Her first bout with cancer was a shock; this time, I don't think we were all that surprised. We can deal with her dying and having cancer, but it's watching her suffer that is the worst. She unfortunately has a grim prognosis and will probably get worse and will not last more than a year, if that.

"Emotionally, in all three cases the only way we dealt/deal with it was/is through a lot of faith and prayer. We support each other and try to help each other cope with watching the progression of the disease(s). We talk about it often, I guess in a way to desensitize ourselves to it. The hardest part for us has been being related to them. I would have liked to just play the role of the son to my father, turning over the caregiving responsibility to those who are trained to do so by profession. I don't like to admit it but there was a bit of resentment on both my wife's and my parts because of the burden placed on us. Of course, we had guilt because of feeling this way, but we are only human, and it is very difficult being a caregiver, especially also being disabled. It would have been a lot less emotional and easier if we could detach ourselves from the situation(s), but of course, we couldn't do that since they are our own flesh and blood.

"We feel things are best for my father-in-law and my dad. They are in a far better place and no longer suffer. With my mom, we will have to see. As my mom is the only one we are caring for now, we know we will watch her get progressively worse and we will have to give more and more care until she goes home to God, as well."

Barbara's Story

"In my late 30s, I began feeling like something was missing in my life. But I was not sure what it was. I also kept wondering if there was more to life, and how I would go about finding out what that was for me.

"In late 2004 my chocolate Lab, Cassie, was diagnosed with terminal bone cancer. Watching her live with cancer as if each day was still the same really opened me up to wanting to live my own days with more joy. Not that I didn't enjoy my life, but I wanted to do something more meaningful. I started to wonder what my legacy would be. Would people even know I was here, someday? This led me to hire a life coach to help me dive down into my heart and discover what it was that brought me joy, and then in turn help me start living in that way.

"After three months of coaching, I was on top of the world. I decided to pursue writing, and writing about my favorite subject – dogs. As I was on my way to doing just this, nine months later my Dachshund, Frankie, was diagnosed with Intervertebral Disc Disease (IVDD). I knew nothing about the disease, which causes degeneration of the discs and sometimes they rupture. One of Frankie's discs ruptured from a fall, which caused paralysis in her hind legs.

181

"After being rushed to the veterinary hospital that would do surgery, I was given only a 10% guarantee that she would walk on her own again. There was a real possibility she would not regain the use of her back legs.

"I was devastated. I couldn't imagine how she could live a quality life without the use of her legs. I had never seen a dog in this condition before. I also went through feeling very mad that I was being handed this. I questioned whether or not I really wanted to take care of a handicapped dog.

"From all of this, it actually led to my calling and my purpose. I knew I wanted to educate others about this disease, as so often if people are not educated, the pet is put to sleep. It is a disease that does not have a cure, but dogs can live full, long quality lives even with IVDD. Through taking Frankie out in public, I also realized she was having a positive effect on children, helping them see their own challenges in a positive way.

"This led me to write a children's book series about Frankie. For four years we visited local schools and libraries in my state of Wisconsin. Frankie also became a certified therapy dog and we made over 250 visits to a local hospice, hospital and senior assisted living facility. Those were honestly, so far, the best years of my life – even though I couldn't imagine at the beginning of the ordeal that it would all turn out this way.

"I was finally stepping into my truth and authenticity. I learned to accept myself for who I was. The key thing for me was having a dog in a wheelchair, which taught me this. At first, I was scared others would think I was cruel or mean for doing this. But I know in my heart how happy Frankie is – she has a full, quality life. Who cares what others think? I thought one day. It was then that I

realized that about myself. To just live my life the best I can, and the way I want to live it – and not worry how others think I should live my life – it was so freeing for me! Today, I am just not the same person I was before this all happened. I'm so much stronger. I love living in my own skin. I love being me. I stand strong in who I am and what I believe. I'm much more compassionate and I am so much more open to life. And all because of a little love dog on wheels!"

B eing a caregiver for someone who has been afflicted with illness or some other life-altering circumstance comes with its own set of challenges, as well as its rewards. First, the person being cared for (the survivor) may not be the same person as before, mentally, physically or emotionally. Often, his or her abilities and behaviors may be substantially different, and the caregiver has to learn how to cope with these changes, as if mourning the loss of the loved one who doesn't exist anymore.

Instead of looking at what the survivor's life was once like, it may be necessary to look forward and create a new and different story based on his or her current situation. For example, he may have been a scientist like Lynn's husband or an engineer like Suzanne's husband, or an avid runner completing multiple-mile marathons, or she may have traveled to exotic places around the world. But now, they may be restricted by their conditions, so the "story" must change.

It's times like these when one starts to see that the simplest pleasures in life can be more precious than the biggest, most elaborate life plans that one considers important. Instead of running miles, where the focus is on the outcome of the race, a simple walk together in the park allows for intimate conversation and communing with one's surroundings, an activity that may be more heartfelt and meaningful. Lynn and her husband have worked as a team to come up with options to accommodate his limited mobility, such as his iPad, which keeps him in touch with the world so he can continue to exercise his scientific mind. Maybe if she can't travel to some fascinating spot across the globe, she can bring it home like Sue did in "What if I Don't Fully Recover?" Remember the Caribbean vacation she took in the comfort of her own home? The caregiver needs to find activities that are of interest and that can be done within the new life framework. It's about living in the present and enjoying each moment as it comes.

This isn't always easy for the caregiver, just as it isn't always easy for the survivor. The caregiver may go through a grieving process, much like the survivor does. The first stage is shock at what has happened to the loved one's physical, mental and/or emotional condition. Then there's the sadness as the caregiver grieves over the loss of how their charge used to be. And finally, the caregiver goes through his or her own recovery by accepting the current situation and moving forward with a new story. To help one get through this period (which may last weeks, months, years or indefinitely) and not feel so alone as a caregiver, joining a support group would have similar benefits to those for the survivor, to have an established support system in place. Seek one at a local hospital or at one of the various online caregiver resources pertinent to the survivor's condition.

One of the biggest but most rewarding challenges for the caregiver is to change one's perception. Although one's charge may no longer be the person of the past, it's important to see what he or she has to offer now in their present form: the strength they still have, the positivity they can offer, even if it's as small as a smile or kind gesture or word. And even in the face of adversity – the belligerent behavior, the physical or emotional lashing out – the caregiver can gain an inner strength that comes from seeking the silver lining on the darkest of clouds, by seeing one not as a victim of circumstance, but as a servant of one's own soul and of the universe. Several of the caregivers from this chapter used their experiences to share their messages of help and healing in their own individual ways.

We all have our place in the world, our purpose in life; and as we are faced with life situations that shake us to the core, we find that these times of distress and hardship can actually empower us and elevate us to a higher level of character. We may become a whole different person, whereas in the past, we may have been a person concerned only with our material life and our big dreams of how we would like our life to be. And there's nothing wrong with that, in the relative world! But often, we lose sight of the little things that are so meaningful and can spark the flames of an inner abundance that can prevail over our outer world proclivities.

From what can we derive small pleasures? What are the small moments that can bring us joy and happiness in the new life set before us? This is what we should shoot for!

EXERCISE

In your journal or notebook, make two columns. In the left column, write down the activities your charge used to do in life. In the right column, write down a substitute activity for each one that you can do with your charge now. Do this with your charge, so that you both come up with a plan for creating a new "story" for the new life that awaits you both. And don't forget – as a caregiver, please find the support you need. You may be the caregiver, but you need just as much support as your charge does.

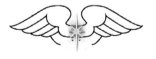

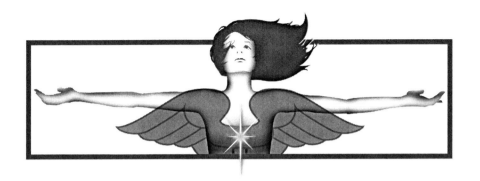

Lessons Learned
and Pearls of Wisdom

"Your life will be transformed into something very different to what it was before...your beliefs, your thoughts, your values, your behavior, your actions. You will become a whole new person, and what kind of person will depend on how you deal with your recovery emotionally."

As you know, before I had my stroke, I was working 80 hours a week. I held a corporate management position in a Fortune 500 company. I was also trying to get my healing arts business off the ground, and I was publishing two books I had authored. I was leading a full life, to say the least, and actually enjoying what I was doing, albeit I was exhausted most of the time.

When I had my stroke, I was forced to get off the fast-paced treadmill of life and start moving at a snail's pace. Boy, did my life change dramatically! The early days and months after my stroke were spent doing rehab and sleeping, and not much more. It was as if I was catching up on years of pushing myself, as my body demanded hours and hours of rest. (I did watch a lot of TV, though. The Hallmark channel became my fantasy world!) I'm sure you can imagine how I felt going from the hectic hare-like life that I had pre-stroke, to the slow tortoise-like life post-stroke. But during my recovery, I began to luxuriate in my new unhurried life, and I learned so much about how a traumatic life situation can really transform a person in so many ways.

Where I had been so impatient before, I learned to accept that things would happen in their own Divine time, without me pushing them to happen according to my schedule. Where I had been driven by aggression and the need to control, I was able to surrender to my inner Divine guidance, which was grounded in heart-consciousness. I began to identify my limiting beliefs, which prevented me from having the abundance that was my birthright. I'm not talking just about material abundance. I'm talking about the emotional abundance one feels when they are fulfilling their deepest desires, in alignment with what Spirit wants for them as their destiny. To repeat my mantra: "I'm on a magic carpet ride, with Spirit at the helm." I began to see what was really important in life. It wasn't about my outer reality, the material things I had that were indicators of success. It wasn't about how much I was recognized by others. These are good things to have, but they only feed the ego. They don't nourish the soul.

I found that seeking my inner essence and having a loving relationship with myself were what really validated my place in the world. From this heart center, I could radiate love out into the world, which would touch other people's lives. That is where true success and abundance are, in my eyes. These are but a few of the lessons I learned from having a stroke. It truly was a gift from the soul.

Now read about the lessons that were learned by the story contributors of this book, as they all had their own unique "ah-ha" moments springing from their situations.

Survivors

Aurelio: "My heart is now softer and gentler after allowing myself the experience of feeling all the hurt, anger, and terror that I had suppressed for most of my life."

Callie: "The overwhelming feeling that my life was meant to be lived as a joyfully loving experience, through laughter and play, saw me taking time out and restructuring my entire life – and my business – to support my new vision of life."

Cindy: "Living with a chronic illness for the past 20 years has helped me grow in many different ways I never thought possible. I greet each new day with a more appreciative grace, I can find love in places I never thought possible and I am filled with gratitude."

Cherry-Lee: "I learned I was truly able to trust myself and my intuition, even if it didn't feel like it at each moment. It empowered me for my later pregnancy, when I was able to speak my truth and hold with it until people listened. Once Avalon (my first-born) was born, and I had had my near-death-experience, I found that the veils between worlds were thin. I became a regular meditator for the first time ever. It took about a year for my vision to return so that I could read. When it did, I learned about the tarot and read extensively on spirituality. I had dreams and kept a journal. The whole world became alive for me daily in a way that I had only previously experienced during high moments."

Deny: "One cannot be completely well unless one's body, mind and spirit are healed. When one suffers, the others suffer as well.

"Your health (body, mind and spirit) is all that matters. Everything else is superfluous. Every day, practice activities that will bring health to your body, mind and spirit.

"Truly give thanks every day for all of the blessings in your life. There are more than you may think."

Joe: "I've learned recovery truly is a process, and there were quite a few steps involved for me. Forgiveness was probably the most critical. I wasn't able to begin to heal until I forgave my abuser. I never blamed my parents for missing the signs, but for my own sake, I forgave them as well. Trust and courage were very important and went hand-in-hand. I found the courage to talk about what happened and the ability to trust someone with the whole truth.

"Restoring my faith in God has been the latest step. The realization that through Him I can turn my mess into a message to help others was a huge step. I went through what I went through for a reason. I'm still going through the process, even 20-some years after the abuse ended. Every time I share my story, I recover a little bit more. Every time I listen to someone who is somewhere along that road, I recover a little bit more."

Katherine: "I learned a practical spirituality, which I can apply to every aspect of my life. I choose a life that is about receiving and communicating love and the innocence we share in God."

Kim: "I learned that before you can do anything for God, family or anyone really, you must take care of yourself. We women have a tendency not to take the time to eat, sleep or exercise to keep our body going, to accomplish the things God has [in store] for us."

Pamina: "I learned not to underestimate the power of our parental relating patterns; how deeply they are imprinted in our psyches. Despite consciously vowing that repeating these is as desirable as developing bleeding hemorrhoids, the chances are high that we will end up duplicating exactly what we don't want – or slamming the pendulum so far over the other way that this damages us just as badly. The drive to repeat the familiar, combined with the equally powerful drive to create an opposite reality, lays a very confusing trap into which I, along with many others, fell.

"Laughing at my own idiocy has granted me a finely tuned crap alarm. Having developed an ability to identify mine instantly, decoding the patterns in others is second nature. Living my mission with finely honed navigational skills empowers me to negotiate life from the driver's seat with confidence and clarity. I instinctively sense the potholes and multiple pile-ups. The accumulated skills of a lifetime and well-developed intuition enable me to pursue my dreams and expand my fear fences. I'm not afraid to look like a fool. I know there's no such thing as failure; that physically, emotionally and mentally I will always survive; and that I'm infinitely valuable.

"Becoming a writer has built my immunity to rejection beyond my wildest dreams. I thoroughly recommend it! Feeling the sting of rejection is a certainty in life. But rejection is only an opinion and I refuse to allow rejection to cripple or define me."

Sabine: "Never take tomorrow for granted. Don't put off the things you want to do in life, because you do not know what the future brings. Be grateful for the things you have, instead of focusing on what you don't have."

Sandi: "There were many lessons that I learned, and continue to learn. The one thing that comes to mind is that all alcoholics drink to change the way they feel. It comes down to that. We are a group of people who normally would not mix, but are bound together by this devastating, uniquely physical, emotional, and spiritual disease. In recovery, I have found a way to live in humility and integrity."

Sue: "I've learnt a few major lessons that only came with time for ME, but the great thing about your book is passing on lessons learnt to others, in a 'this worked for me, try it' kinda way. I learned that it is so important to learn about yourself, what values and beliefs you were brought up with that hold you back, and what works for you. I learned patience (not easy). Things don't happen overnight. I remember feeling so overwhelmed by the enormity of what I felt I had to overcome. Breaking it into bite-sized chunks worked for me (lots of smaller goals)."

Tina: "I was frequently thought of as selfish – I think this behavior was primarily due to having ADD (attention deficit disorder), which went undiagnosed until I was about 38. It wasn't that I was selfish; I was just clueless. It's funny. Now that I'm medicated and much more aware of others' needs, I have had to learn how to be consciously selfish. I never understood (and frankly, was horrified) when the flight attendants would tell passengers to 'secure your oxygen mask first before helping those who may need assistance.' When explained, it was so simple, I felt kind of stupid. If you pass out, how can you help anyone else? I was once told that it was selfish of me NOT to let people help. I find it difficult sometimes to manage all the offers of assistance, but know that others, just as I, likely gain self-worth when they help. On the other hand, beware of those who will martyr themselves in their service of you."

Vanessa: "I learnt about the potential of me, both the positive potential and the negative potential, and how my thoughts had really created my reality. I learnt about balance and honouring myself and my knowing, in every moment."

Caregivers

Barbara: "One of my biggest lessons was finally stepping into my truth and authenticity. I learned to accept myself for who I was. I stopped worrying (for the most part) what others thought of me. Who cares what others think? I thought, one day. To just live my life the best I can, and the way I want to live it – and not worry how others think I should live my life – it was so freeing for me!"

Becki: "Don't take for granted that everything will always be alright, since this has happened to both my mother and her sister. I now have systems in place, should things like this happen to me. My husband has both legal and medical Power of Attorney for me, so that he and my children do not have to worry about the things I went through with my mom."

Bob: "I feel that most people are too proud or don't know where to get help. You have to swallow your pride and seek help for you as a caregiver, and for your loved one. If I could redo this part of my life, I'd set up the contact lists before things got really bad. Always be proactive in life, for we never think it will happen to us; and when it does, it can be frightening. I also feel that to be an effective caregiver, you must take care of yourself while you're caregiving. You'll find if you don't care for yourself, you'll have a very hard time caring for your loved one. I myself focused on my father, who suffered a severe stroke, and got very sick. Later, I learned to take care of myself, so Dad would be properly cared for."

Erica: "I have learned to be grateful for little things. I have remembered how powerful the human spirit can be if you truly believe you can accomplish things. I have learned that we all possess internal strengths that often need to be fostered and nurtured to realize their true potential."

Lynn: "Caregiving has taught me that each new day is a gift, an opportunity to do good and to make the best of each situation. It has made me appreciate people and good health, and shown me the importance of taking good care of both. Dad's passing simplified life for me, giving me a better perspective of what is truly important. Showing those whom we hold dear just how special they are to us while they are still on this Earth is paramount! Let's not wait for a funeral to show our love and kindness for others!"

Mark: "Patience. Recovery from stroke, in its myriad forms, takes time. It does not come quickly or instantly."

Michael: "You find you can do a lot more than you think you can, when caring for someone you love. I also learned that if you can have [an external] caregiver instead of you being the caregiver, then that would be best. Take for instance my dad. It would have been better for me to remain in the role of son, rather than any part of the role of caregiver. Even the folks from the hospice told us we should have remained in our natural roles, rather than taking on being caregivers. Of course, we continue to do it, but I do not recommend it for others. You have to evaluate a lot of things in your life before taking on that role."

Suzanne: "I learned to have more compassion and patience; to understand what people deal with when a family member is disabled; to understand what it means to be a caregiver; to understand how disability affects a family; that I am stronger than I believed I was; that I could do things I didn't think I could, such as taking care of a disabled person's needs of bathing, feeding, bathroom, shower, etc., as well as trying to support them emotionally, physically and spiritually; that I had a bigger purpose through a major life challenge; that life can be very difficult but there is still laughter, joy and love and that is what makes all the difference; how strong and amazing my children were through this and how they have grown to be strong, compassionate loving people, probably even more because of this experience, and how much they loved their father.

"At times I felt like I was the caterpillar in the chrysalis. It was dark and scary and questions came to mind like 'Now what?' 'What's next?' and 'What am I supposed to do?' Just like the caterpillar, we don't realize there is a bigger purpose in this darkness. Through this darkness, we can spread our wings. We can become this beautiful butterfly full of grace and beauty. What does it take for this caterpillar to turn into the beautiful butterfly? It takes trust, patience and an inner knowing that something powerful and beautiful is about to transpire. This is how I see the journey and this is why even on the darkest days, there is an inner knowing that despite it all, it will be alright and I will be a more empowered being, just like the butterfly."

All of the story contributors learned different things based on their circumstances, as you will learn things based on your own experiences. One thing that I feel for sure will happen as you go through your recovery is your life will be transformed into something very different to what it was before...your beliefs, your thoughts, your values, your behavior, your actions. You will become a whole new person, and what kind of person will depend on how you deal with your recovery emotionally.

I wish to close the book with some pearl of wisdom that I hope will help keep your spirits uplifted. I will include mine and those of the story contributors. As for mine, I will simply repeat the themes in the book, as they played a huge role in my healing.

- Never give up
- Believe in yourself
- Have gratitude for what you have in your life

- Keep a good attitude, as much as possible
- Squelch any limiting beliefs that prevent you from being who you should be
- Know that you are co-creators with Spirit, who will never lead you astray
- Surround yourself with a good support system of friends, family and, of course, your own inner support
- Understand that recovery is a process and it takes several steps, so be patient with yourself
- Live in the present, to enjoy every precious moment of life
- And finally, know what's really important in life

Of course, the story contributors have their own pieces of advice that they wanted to share.

Survivors

Deny: "Never give up! Through suffering comes enlightenment. Use it to change your life."

Aurelio: "Love yourself first! It all starts with loving and accepting yourself. It's so easy to say and yet so difficult to do. But that is where all true healing starts."

Callie: "Okay. So now we know what we are dealing with...what do you wish to let go of, so you can really embrace all the goodness in your life? I would also strongly recommend art therapy – it saved my sanity and helped me dream big, bold and beautiful ideas that I am now living! Just reach out, connect with others and know – beyond ANY shadow of a doubt – that you are loved and gloriously perfect in your imperfection."

Sandi: "If I had one thing to tell others facing similar challenges, I would simply share my story. I would talk about my experience, strength, and hope with him or her so they could see that they are not alone. We have more similarities than differences. Going to a recovery center and being an alcoholic/addict is not a stigma or something to be ashamed of, but a disease. Recovery offers a life that you never thought possible – a life of spirit and spirituality without using the wrong spirits."

Kim: "Don't give up or give in. Find what you need, who you need and drastically change your thinking."

Pamina: "Embrace change and live in the moment; be flexible and adapt to a variety of environments and circumstances. Knowing how quickly and unexpectedly those you love can disappear from your life, increase the intensity of your love and appreciation."

Vanessa: "Honor yourself in every moment!"

Cherry-Lee: "Be open to miracles and listen to the first nudge – don't wait for the big ones! Trust that inner voice and the messages you get from your body!"

Cindy: "To someone who has just been diagnosed with MS, I would say, "Do not let this become your death sentence." You are stronger than you think and this life challenge you have been given is simply a roadblock for you to become fearless. Be positive, be powerful and smile a secret smile."

Joe: "If something is not right, have the courage to speak up. Find someone you can trust with the truth and don't be afraid of the consequences. You'll be amazed at how brave you can be."

Katherine: "Hang in there. You are more beautiful and more important than you know."

Sue: "Learn about yourself, learn how you tick. Learn about your new values and beliefs, what works for you now that's different to what it was before. Are you doing things for yourself or for others? Get in contact with your new identity."

Sabine: "Focus on what you have left, and not on what you have lost. Focus on a positive outcome, and truly believe in that. That focus will give you the strength you need to not give up."

Tina: "Don't be a whiney-ass victim! Yes, we are all entitled to a pity party now and again, but I recommend you 1) announce what you are doing to anyone who needs to know, 2) have it ALONE (maybe with a pint of Blue Bell) and 3) really wallow in it – sob, sputter snot boogers, wail, moan or scream, "Why? Why? Why?" while looking at yourself in the mirror until you can't help but laugh at yourself. Then remember the reason it is you is because you can handle it when no one else around you could. Blow your nose, splash your face and rejoin the rest of the world."

Caregivers

Barbara: "First of all, never give up hope. Second, I would say, take the time to be still each and every day and really listen to what your heart and soul are trying to tell you. I think so often we truly do have the answer for our lives, but we get caught up in what society thinks or says we should do. But more often than not, we really do know the answer. It is fear that gets in the way of living the life we truly want to live. But I can say that once you start living your life the way you want, you will never want to live it any other way."

Becki: "Don't take for granted that everything will always be alright."

Bob: "Being a caregiver is very rewarding, but you'll never face more pressure in your life as you do as a caregiver! The way to deal with this is to be positive, as this will transfer to your loved one. Your loved one is highly dependent on you and will pick up on everything you do or feel. The way to divert this problem is for the caregiver and loved one to get involved in positive diversions in life. This can be watching comedies, listening to pleasant music, joining a church/club, walking, attending family gatherings, or anything else that develops positive feelings between all of you."

Erica: "How you choose to view the event is all you – although you cannot control the event itself (or disease or illness), you can control how you view it. Perspective makes a huge difference and I know that looking for the good in the situation is a helpful strategy. My mom has given me a good piece of advice on this, too. When I get frustrated by Jim's actions (or lack of actions), she reminds me, "It is the illness, Erica. It's not Jim." I think coming up with a phrase that you can tell yourself when you want to scream because everything is so frustrating and unfair will help. Besides my mother's phrase, I tell myself often, "Believe." This helps. So simple, but so powerful."

Lynn: "Explore the options and resources that are available. Keep searching for a reasonable solution until you find one that works for you. Take care of yourself in order to continue providing quality and compassionate care to your loved one, without sacrificing your own wellbeing. Choose to succeed, instead of accepting the status quo or feeling like a victim. You have the ability within you to create a positive atmosphere and to choose a positive outlook, to accomplish what you need to accomplish. Don't let obstacles stop you, but challenge yourself to find a way around them!"

Mark: "Try to remember it is not the fault of the person that they had a stroke. They did not choose this path."

Michael: "If you have the opportunity to obtain an external caregiver and remain in your natural familial role, then do so."

Suzanne: "Even on the darkest and most challenging of days, trust that there is a higher purpose to it all, even if you don't feel it. Spirit is always with you and all is well. Close your eyes and let your inner guidance answer your questions and concerns."

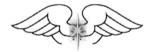

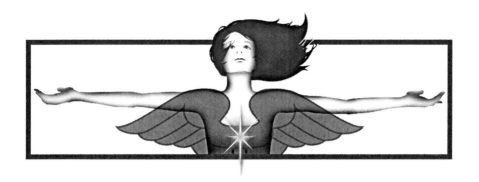

Coming Full Circle

"How we respond to the adversities of life will dictate whether we rise up out of the ashes like the invincible phoenix or sink into a mire of hopelessness."

E aster weekend, followed by my birthday on April 2, was a very important time for me. That was the time in which I began to come "full circle" in my recovery from my stroke. It's interesting to me that Easter was so close to my birthday this year, as if the "resurrection" and my birth (or should I say, my rebirth or transformation of self) coincided.

I felt like I went through my own form of crucifixion, as the few weeks that led up to this very significant time were gruesome, yet extraordinary. As I went through this period, I kept in my journal all that happened and all that went through my mind, and I wish to share it with you to see how it all culminated in my "resurrection." I will reveal the details that had the most relevance.

The first night that things started getting hairy, I was in bed trying to sleep, but then the anxieties started – anxieties I thought I had overcome – and they were severe. I started thinking about committing suicide, and I wondered why that morbid thought had entered my mind. Then I remembered the past life that was related to my stroke, where I saw the "symbolic" hole in my heart and how I had killed myself due to lost love. I must have been replaying those feelings of wanting to die in my head.

As you might remember, that was the love of the same man I dearly loved once again in this lifetime. The man so near and dear to my heart was not only special to me on the physical plane in this lifetime, but on the spiritual plane as well. As an "emissary of the gods," he helped my femininity emerge. I discuss this in my novel *Anything Is Possible*. The following passage is a synthesis of text from the book *Sacred Prostitute* by the Jungian analyst Nancy Qualls-Corbett.

"She was the sacred prostitute [who became a spiritually empowered woman, as opposed to the 'profane prostitute' who was debased...awaiting her patron's arrival], proceeding through an ancient ritual of the maiden, through the reverence of the Goddess Venus, being empowered with her natural feminine sexuality. The ritual was that of a 'stranger,' identified as an emissary of the gods, appearing before the maiden, and through their intimate encounter, she would be transformed...into a woman very much connected to her inner femininity. The stranger was unexpected, uninvited and of 'foreign nature.'"28

He was the "foreign stranger" who came into my life unexpectedly and initiated my transformation of self, where I would become connected with my inner femininity. He also represented the positive masculine energy within (driving outward manifestation, highly focused, goal-oriented and ambitious) that was to come back to life eventually, washing away the negative dark side of the masculine energy (aggression, control and domination). This made perfect sense, as he was so very focused on the outer world, always achieving the goals he set for himself.

Through this man's love, while the negative masculine energy inside me was dismantled, the positive masculine energy awakened. My feminine side emerged, taking it by the hand and leading it down the path to unity. As I paraphrase what I said in "My Story" and which has been the theme throughout this book, "The feminine determines what is to be created, then engages the masculine to manifest this creation into being, thus creating inner stasis, with the Yin and Yang working in harmony." The one cannot be without the other. This unity is synonymous with love, the love that exists within, at the heart level, and radiates outwardly at the physical level, into the world. If this love is hindered in any way, there can be no inner harmony.

This inner harmony was further expressed in a class I took on polarity energy balancing to renew my massage license. "If love is blocked, life force will be blocked, and the body will reflect this."[29] Polarity energy balancing is a simple and effective method to bring deep healing relaxation by using the life force currents (a subtle form of electromagnetic energy) that naturally flow through everyone's hands. This life force is called by many names – chi or ki, the light, prana, orgone energy – to name a few. The principle behind polarity is balancing the opposites. Sound familiar?

The body has similar electromagnetic charges, just like the Earth's magnetic field has + (positive) and – (negative) charges at the North Pole and South Pole, respectively. The top (the head) and the right side are positive; the bottom (the feet) and left side are negative. Blocked areas within this natural energy field cause imbalances that are manifested as physical or (emotional) ailments. Polarity energy balancing treats these imbalances, balancing the electromagnetic field, recharging the life force in a person. This results in a relaxation of the nerves, which can lead to significant changes, both physically and emotionally. I found it very intriguing that this was one of the classes I chose to take at this time to renew my license, which expired at the end of April (my birth month). Just one more way of emphasizing my need for inner balance, for my full healing.

I realized something else as I pondered this inner balance that I had been working on so extensively. I had pushed myself in the 5K run at the end of 2012. Though it was a milestone, showing me what I could do, I did it with the old masculine mindset and, of course, the therapists at the rehab center who put me on the road to my full recovery were also pushing me to make it to the end. While it may have been good that I finished the run, was it really good for my full healing, considering I was trying to shift away from the spirit of force and muscle and move into the light of surrender?

My body was a reflection that I was not balanced...still trying, but not quite there yet! And for the one-and-a-half weeks before Easter, my body seemed to take a turn for the worse. My right side stopped working almost completely, as if I was reverting back to the way I was when I first had my stroke. I couldn't even go to rehab or do my home exercises because my body wouldn't let me. As I delved deep into my soul to find some answers to why this was happening, I received a very clear message: "You must surrender completely!" Then I remembered a meditation I had practiced almost exactly one year before. Fortunately, I had written it down in my journal, so I had most of the details.

"Image of queen ant on the left side of my body, as if on a podium directing a colony of ants on the right side of my body. The ant is a symbol of work and industry. The laborer ants doing all of the work are female (I was asking the left side to help heal my right side). The ant is an architect, a teacher of how you become an architect of your own life, being patient with your efforts and yourself. The queen dies after 12 years. In numerology, 12 = 3, which is the number of my birthday. This cycle of 12 years is significant regarding the building of goals. The ant teaches that regardless of the circumstances, if the effort is true, rewards will follow in the most beneficial time and manner. The queen ant was telling her laboring force of female ants to work with the nerves of my right side to innervate the muscles."

When I associated this meditation on its one-year anniversary with the message I received about surrender, it was so clear what it all meant. I had to truly let go of the masculine ethos of taking action and just allow myself to be in that passive state, being guided by Spirit, and by doing so, "the rewards [would] follow in the most beneficial time and manner" as my meditation indicated.

What was going on in mind, body and spirit was a reflection of me getting closer to my resurrection. The intensity of the feelings I was having was an indication that I was clearing out all the karma related to my stroke and thus moving into that place of inner balance, where the masculine and feminine elements of my psyche frolicked together. Even the thoughts of suicide that flitted about in my head were simply expressions of the old ways of thinking "dying," making way for the new. It was my transformation of self. I was "coming full circle" in my life.

Then on April 4, four days after Easter and two days after my birthday, I was discharged from rehab. I was shocked because I didn't think I was ready for it. But when my occupational and physical therapists evaluated me, they said my strength was incredible. I just had to work on my endurance. So they sent me home with exercises to add to my existing home exercise program and told me to come back in two months for a re-evaluation. At first, I was sad. I had been there for almost two years through my recovery. It was like my home away from home. Now I was on my own to finish out my recovery.

But then I had a mind shift! I realized I felt that my full recovery would go more swiftly after being released from rehab because being in rehab made me feel that I was "sick." Being out of rehab gave me the unconscious message that I wasn't sick anymore. So now, I would just go about my business as if I were well – because I WAS WELL!

Another mind shift happened almost simultaneously. When I first started writing this book, I was about 85% recovered and saying that I hoped I would be 100% recovered by the time I finished it. That hope, I felt, came from my old ethos of wanting to control everything and expecting it to happen when I wanted it to; thus, it was a false hope.

Now you may be asking, "What's wrong with having hope? Hasn't the aim of this book been to offer hope to others?" Yes, yes, very, very true! But for me, I had always lived in the mode of controlling everything in my life. And as I continued writing, each chapter bringing to light the issues I needed to work on as I moved through my metamorphosis during my recovery, I got further from the spirit of control and expectations to one of surrender, again moving from the masculine to the feminine; from the place of action to the place of letting go; and then to that heart-centered place of being, where that inner sense of harmony that I so desire is. Or so I thought.

For the next several weeks, I went through yet another phase of conflict between control and letting go. My body went through another downturn, but even worse than before. It was as if I was spiraling out of control. My right limbs had no strength or stability. Whereas I had begun walking and jogging just weeks before, now I could barely walk around the house, and my arm and hand began to feel like they were no longer part of my body. What was going on *this* time? Maybe spiraling out of control was a good thing. Maybe this was the very last leg of my journey. It had been the roller coaster ride of my life and I really was tired of all the valleys I was passing through.

It's been said in so many ways that "it's when you've reached the end of your rope that the miracle happens." And I was at my wits' end. But once again, I had to surrender all expectations.

I knew my full recovery from my stroke would come and I would no longer feel that I had to put a date or time when it would happen, as it's being Divinely guided. And what was really fascinating to me was that I decided to return not to my salsa lessons, but to my ballet lessons, to finish out my recovery – and the studio where I was going to take those lessons was the one where I did my very first "plié" as a young girl.[30] And it's uncanny that the studio has moved only a mile from where I live. Talk about "coming full circle"! My metamorphosis was almost complete. Someday I would break out of my chrysalis and, as a butterfly stretches its new wings, fly free of the encumbrances of my mind and allow Spirit to continue to work through me.

Life is replete with ebbs and flows. The tides will bring us times of great joy and hope, but just as easily wash it all away. We are challenged each day so that we may grow into our own personal power. But how we respond to the adversities will dictate whether we rise up out of the ashes like the invincible phoenix or sink into a mire of hopelessness.

Look at your life right now. Yes, you may be facing serious misfortune, but what can you do to turn what you may consider the worst affliction in your life into a treasure brimming with pearls of wisdom and lessons learned? Life is meant to be good, so how can you transform your life from one of despair to one of hope and radiance?

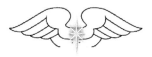

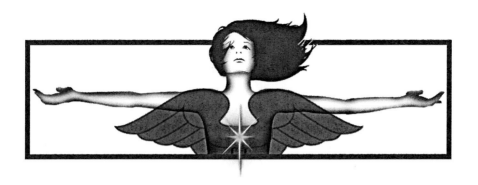

The Beginning of
My New Life

> *"No matter how long it takes to recover and heal from any life-altering experience, we should all see our journey as a 'magic carpet ride with Spirit at the helm' – and if we really believe in ourselves, we can 'watch the miracles unfold.'"*

It was the end of June 2013. My journey of recovery and healing wasn't over, but I could feel in my heart that July was going to be the awakening of a new life full of love, joy and harmony. My journey thus far had been a ride full of twists and turns but I felt that from here on out, the road would be less bumpy. I would be like a butterfly, free from the hindrances of any fears that would raise their ugly heads and try to pull me into a chasm of despair.

I saw that the timing for my release from rehab had been in perfect Divine order. I had to go through the descent into the total darkness of my psyche, where the sacred fires were burning away the residue of my karma. On the physical level, the right side of my body felt as if it had regressed. My leg, particularly my foot, had little sensation and was very weak, as if it wasn't even there. My right arm just dangled from my shoulder with very little strength or stability. Spirit had tested me to the nth degree.

I had to trust that I would be completely healed, that I, like the phoenix, would rise from the ashes victorious. I had done my part and now it was time to really "let go and let God." Yes, I've said this time and time again, but surrendering was so very hard for me. Yet if I wanted to brush off the debris from the fires that had extinguished my suffering so that I could spread my wings and fly to freedom, it was a must.

And my dreams reflected my progress. One night I had a dream of light around me and a sense of peace, indicating to me that I was in the arms of Spirit. Another night I dreamed of townhouses, beautiful upscale townhouses similar to the ones I was actually looking to move into, when I was well enough. The only room I visited in my dream was the bathroom, which is representative of our need to cleanse ourselves, removing waste via the toilet and emerging purified through bathing. I gathered that this was a reflection of what I was going through, a cleansing of my soul.

And the message that I was ALMOST THERE rang out loud and clear when a very dear friend with considerable psychic powers came to visit for a weekend and gave me a magical reading that confirmed both the success of my recovery and what I had to look forward to in the future. She said that because of the work I had already done – the therapy and exercise – my physical body was actually already healed. Remember in "Coming Full Circle" when I mentioned that because I was discharged from rehab, I felt I was no longer sick, that I was well instead? What I was going through was the spiritual part of the healing process that was causing the unusual dysfunction of my body, and one day I would wake up and my body would be alive again. It had everything to do with my commitment to surrendering. When I "let go and let God," my healing would be complete.

And as grace would have it, a day after my friend returned home, she emailed me to tell me about a sermon she was listening to by Joel Osteen, the senior minister at Lakewood Church in Houston. You may remember me mentioning him previously. He was telling the story of one of his parishioners, a 50-something-year-old man who had had a stroke and for two years was wheelchair-bound, totally paralyzed on his left side, and he couldn't talk. The doctors said there was no hope for recovery. Then miraculously, one day, he woke up and felt sensation on his paralyzed side.

Osteen went on to say that today, you would never know this man had a stroke. He walks without a glitch and his speech is perfect. It was the power of prayer and the man's faith that he would recover that caused this miracle to happen. And this, my dear friend said, would happen to me as I continued to surrender to the Divine. There is a plaque on the ceiling above my massage therapist's table that says, "The power that created the body can heal the body." What could be more appropriate to my situation?

And as I patiently waited for my "physical" miracle, the most amazing things happened. I was blessed with several other miracles within a few days of each other that pertained to this book, which I consider as much a part of my healing as my physical recovery, since I wrote it from my heart and wish to spread the radiance of its messages to as many people as possible. And I was graced with the opportunity to do just that because of articles I had written for some wonderfully inspirational websites that had audiences of "millions" of people worldwide. I was also graced with the agreement from some phenomenal people, who were also radiant survivors, to provide testimonials for my book, as well as those willing to participate in my 3-day telesummit that would form part of my book launch. My dream of being able to touch the lives of many people who had gone through or were going through their own life challenges was starting to come true.

And my plan to return to rehab starting July 1, after three months of being off, would help me make the final physical shift in my transformation. I felt that this time I would be operating from my heart-centered, more nurturing mindset. Instead of relentlessly pushing myself as I had done before, I would be gentler on myself. I would create the inner balance of the masculine and feminine principles, that inner unity I so desired to make my transformation complete. Would my physical miracle happen then? Only time and faith would tell.

My story could go on and on, since every day brings something new and exciting. Although I had hoped that physically I would be completely recovered by the time I finished writing my book, I realized it was more important to be healed at the soul level, in communion with my own inner divinity. And I knew that my body would completely heal because I had surrendered to that divinity. No matter how long it takes to recover and heal from any life-altering experience, we should all see our journey as a "magic carpet ride with Spirit at the helm" – and if we really believe in ourselves, we can "watch the miracles unfold."

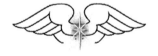

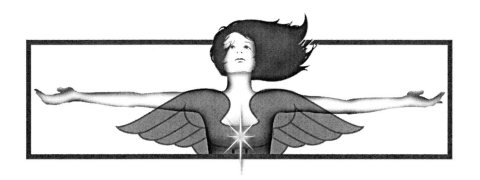

Closing Words

I hope you enjoyed reading *Radiant Survivor* and that you derived some benefit from its messages during your time of recovery and healing. I feel that my story is your story, as we make our way down our path to our new radiant lives. We have been presented with an opportunity to take our life-altering experiences and choose to let them either propel us forward on a journey of inner peace or make us sink in the quicksand of despair. I determined I wasn't going to sink! And I hope you've chosen the same for yourself. I would like to close by summarizing the missives imparted throughout the book, as they bear repeating.

Never underestimate what you can achieve when you believe in yourself! Believing in yourself doesn't come from "with-OUT"; it comes from within, from that heart-centered place where our god/dess essence resides. It's about having self-love. It's about knowing you have something to offer the world – your special gift, whatever it may be. It's about knowing that no matter what your situation is, you have the wherewithal to meet that challenge head on and deal with it.

Life's journey is full of magic – the marvelous, the miraculous and the wonderful – but it's not without its hurdles along the way. And when we come to these bumps in the road, we need to have faith and believe that the Universe "has our back" and will be our pillar of strength, propping us up and propelling us forward. When we surrender to God, the omnipotent, omniscient, and omnipresent power in all of us, magic happens.

When we are in the presence of this inner personal power, we are transformed, and when we are transformed, our world is transformed, because the world is only a reflection, a macrocosm of our microcosm. We are all part of the Divine. And when we are grateful for our blessings and can maintain an optimistic attitude through thick and thin, there's no limit to the opportunities that will present themselves to us.

When one door closes, a new one opens. Life IS meant to be good! Live your life to the fullest, as there is no time to waste! You never know what can happen from one minute to the next, as we have all experienced. Live every precious moment as if it is your last. Then you will have survived and thrived.

And so it is!

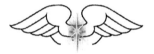

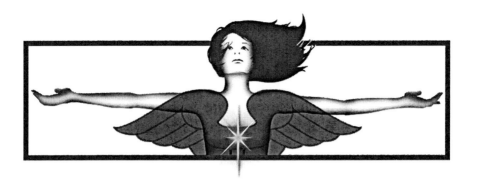

Radiant Survivor (the poem)

Speeding along
On the treadmill of life,
Fell victim to illness
And associated strife.

But Spirit then said
It was a gift of the soul,
Of what you will learn
From a shift in your goals.

Your life will be changed
As you open your heart
To the source of creation,
From which you're never apart.

As you create your new life
You will come to believe
That whatever you do,
You will always achieve.

Never, ever give up
As you strive to recover,
Believe in yourself

And you will discover

That with gracious acceptance
And surrender to the Divine,
Through your treasure from heaven
You're a twinkle in God's eye.

Your situation
Is not who you are.
Change your limiting beliefs
And rise up like a star.

Miracles do happen.
You can shine and thrive
As you lift yourself up
As a Radiant Survivor.

© Erica Tucci February 2013

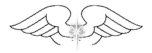

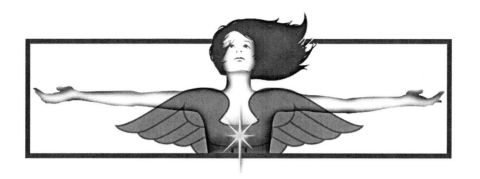

About Author Erica Tucci

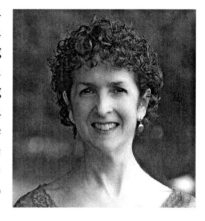

Erica Tucci had a full life as a corporate manager of a Fortune 500 company, a healing arts business owner and an author. It all came to a screeching halt in June 2011 when she had a stroke. Needless to say, her life was changed dramatically. She went from running as fast as she could on the treadmill of life to scooting along at a snail's pace.

During her recovery, she gained much wisdom about what's really important in life and she re-entered the world with a new mission in life. She now wishes to use her story as an inspiration for others facing life challenges, which we all have, big or small. She is developing a trauma recovery coaching program based on her book *Radiant Survivor*. She also wishes to continue the work she was doing before her stroke, helping women find their "yin radiance" through their authentic voice and their own healing. She considers herself the Radiance Muse, inspiring you to live life brilliantly.

For more information, visit www.ericatucci.com and www.radiantsurvivor.com.

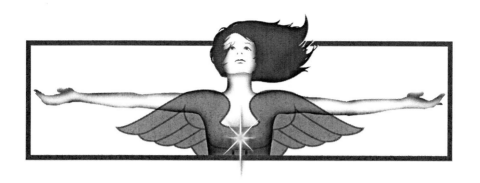

How to Contact
All Story Contributors

Survivors

AURELIO SABLONE, a first-generation Italian-Canadian, was born and raised in Halifax, Nova Scotia. He has a bachelor's degree in Computing Science from Dalhousie University. He is divorced and has joint custody of his beautiful daughter, Aliana. Aurelio is a prolific songwriter and was recently awarded Runner Up placement in the "Song of the Year" contest, a global songwriting competition. His mission is to help others become "raw and radically transparent."

WEB	www.FromGeekToChicTheBook.com
	www.HealYourHeartMusic.com
	www.EZ-GTR.com
FACEBOOK	www.facebook.com/aurelio.sablone
TWITTER	www.twitter.com/AurelioSablone

CALLIE CARLING is the Playfull Genie Muse: a Laughter Yoga teacher, writer, creativity teacher, coach & mentor with boundless energy, Callie is devoted to educating people to cherish and tickle their "playfull" selves, transforming their lives. A breast cancer warrior goddess, she used the 7 Graces as gifts to guide her through her own transformational journey. A lover of decadent afternoon teas, an avid fan of journalling and creating magic with mixed-media, Callie covets vintage china and enjoys playfull adventures in SW London, North Cornwall and Florence, Italy.

WEB	www.createavity.com www.olioterapeutica.co.uk
FACEBOOK	www.facebook.com/moonpoppy www.facebook.com/createavity www.facebook.com/calliecarling
TWITTER	www.twitter.com/moonpoppy
LINKEDIN	www.linkedin.com/in/calliecarling
PINTEREST	www.pinterest.com/moonpoppy

CHERRY-LEE WARD, M.ED. is a contemporary shaman and healer, drawing from traditions around the globe and her inner wisdom. She is an internationally known teacher, mentor and inspiring presenter. Her current passion is to explore the expression of the Sacred Feminine and Masculine in her life and the world around her.

WEB	www.Cherry-LeeWard.com www.cherryleeward.wordpress.com/
FACEBOOK	www.facebook.com/Cherry-Lee Ward
TWITTER	www.twitter.com/Shamanic Healing

CINDY LOTHIAN is a writer, mother and lover of life whose twenty-year dance with the disease MS has taught her that she has multiple strengths. She writes to help bring positivity, confidence, healing, laughter and hope to anyone living with a chronic illness. She is also a columnist at elephantjournal.com and at HuffingtonPost.com and currently working on her own book *Still Sexy after MS*, which she hopes to have published soon.

WEB	www.stillsexyafterms.com
FACEBOOK	www.facebook.com/StillSexyAfterMS
TWITTER	www.twitter.com/sexyafterms

DENY DALLAIRE has survived cancer **six** times. He was even told he had a just a year left to live in 1990. More than 20 years later, and nearly a decade since his last bout of cancer, Deny says that cancer is the best thing that ever happened to him, and that it profoundly changed him for the better. Deny is author of the book: *Many Shades of Green – Running toward the Finish Line, One Cancer at a Time*, and is a much sought-after speaker. His deepest wish is to help everyone achieve their own state of wellness.

FACEBOOK	www.facebook.com/Deny1967 http://goo.gl/Ik6Kr
TWITTER	www.twitter.com/DenyDallaire
LINKEDIN	www.linkedin.com/DenyDallaire

JOE DITTRICH is a survivor of clergy sexual abuse who was featured in the HBO documentary "Priestly Sins: Sex and the Church" in 1996. His recovery has been largely due to counseling and the strength and love of his family and friends. He is still undergoing aspects of emotional, psychological and spiritual growth. He has used his experience to try to support and help others with similar stories. He has rediscovered his faith and is currently on the worship team at his church.

WEB	www.brixenivy.wordpress.com/
FACEBOOK	www.facebook.com/josephdittrich
TWITTER	www.twitter.com/brixen_ivy

KATHERINE T. OWEN pursued spirituality to find peace regardless of the circumstances. She spent 14 years of her life mostly in silence whilst bedbound with severe ME/CFS. Katherine is author of *It's OK to Believe: A Journey with Faith and Reason* and *Be Loved, Beloved*. In *It's OK to Believe*, Katherine takes the reader on a journey to reconcile her questioning mind with her faith. It is a book for all those who have ever asked the big questions about whether we are more than the body.

WEB	www.a-spiritual-journey-of-healing.com
BOOK	www.lulu.com/content/paperback-book/its-ok-to-believe/12383171
FACEBOOK	www.facebook.com/katherine.t.owen
TWITTER	www.twitter.com/spir_jny_heal
LINKEDIN	www.linkedin.com/profile/view?id=83582169
PINTEREST	www.pinterest.com/katherinetowen/

KIM THORNTON is owner and president of Heisreel.com, wife and mother of two. She creates books and films to spread the good news on how to overcome obstacles in life. She has spoken to thousands of people about how to change their lives through the word of God using the only tool she knows: creativity.

WEB	www.Heisreel.com
FACEBOOK	www.facebook.com/Kim Thornton www.facebook.com/Heisreel

TWITTER	www.twitter.com/Heisreel
LINKEDIN	www.linkedin/Heisreel
INSTAGRAM	www.instagram./Heisreel

PAMINA MULLINS, a life coach, hypnotherapist, stress management consultant and writer, spent twenty years in stress survival bootcamp – mostly in Zimbabwe. Her journey through poverty, single parenthood, a child with special needs, bereavement, relocation and divorce made her re-create herself many times over. She now trains others in the art of stress survival, using liberal doses of humour. She is the author of *Why Me?*, *Stress Free You! Unlock Your Emotion Code* and is also a contributing author in *Modern-Day Miracles* by Louise L Hay and Friends.

WEB	www.paminamullins.com
	www.paminamullins.com/blog/
FACEBOOK	www.facebook.com/pamina.mullins

SABINE BECKER was born with very short arms, due to the drug Thalidomide, a so-called "miracle drug" that was prescribed to pregnant women in the late '50s and early '60s to alleviate morning sickness, anxiety and insomnia. Sabine has learned to compensate for her small arms by performing many daily functions and activities with her feet. She is not only a motivational speaker, but also a fund and awareness raiser for disability organizations. In May 2012 she suffered an ischemic stroke. Her whole left side was paralyzed and she lost all fine motor skills in her left foot, which she has used her entire life for daily activities. She also lost her speech, which was especially devastating for her, given that she is a professional public speaker. But through perseverance, determination and a positive outlook, she went from a stroke "victim" to a stroke Survivor.

WEB	www.sabinebecker.org
FACEBOOK	www.facebook.com/sabine.becker2

SANDRA RHEA has her MA in Elementary Education and teaches second grade at Harvard Elementary School in the Houston Heights in Houston, Texas. She has been nominated for Teacher of the Year several times and won this prestigious award on one occasion. She's an aspiring writer and has been published in *Great Educators* and *SAMSHA*. She has overcome overwhelming addictions and is a grateful, recovering alcoholic and food addict. She lives in a sprawling old house in the Houston Heights with her daughter. She loves dogs and cats, children, quilting, teaching, and writing – not necessarily in that order.

FACEBOOK	www.facebook.com/sandra.rhea.35

SUE ROSS survived a major stroke in 1993 and has gone on to retrain as a counselor, life coach and trainer, using her experiences of physical, mental and, most importantly, emotional awareness to impact the lives of others going through the same issues. She founded a group called Lifegeta in 2009, which addresses the emotional issues of people with acquired conditions. She started by running emotional coping workshops, and then monthly meeting groups and a Facebook page where not only the person affected but their family, friends and caregivers can share their experiences.

WEB	www.lifegeta.co.uk
FACEBOOK	www.facebook.com/groups/138794568651

TINA BORJA is a mother of two exceptional teenage boys, a writer, and an editor of academic manuscripts, assorted texts, and non-fiction. Tina's participation in this project was precipitated by the February 12, 2010 diagnosis of Stage 3a invasive ductal carcinoma breast cancer, the February 14, 2012 diagnosis of brain metastasis of the aforementioned, and the fortuitous occasion of her son and the daughter of another guest author falling in love. She believes in magic, that gravity is a collective hallucination, and that cat spit may just be the cure for all illness.

WEB	www.thisposition.wordpress.com

VANESSA BRAGG is a facilitator of vibrational consciousness and social transformation in this era of human awakening. She is an "eternal heart" with an important role to BE in this lifetime. Vanessa is one of the "one people" and helps other eternal hearts energetically access the key to living true potential in changing times. Vanessa is also the creator of The Wisdom Tree.

WEB	www.vanessabragg.com
	www.style2shine.com
	www.thewisdomtree.com.au
FACEBOOK	www.facebook.com/vanessabragg8
TWITTER	www.twitter.com/vanessabragg8

Caregivers

BARBARA TECHEL is an award-winning author of an inspirational memoir *Through Frankie's Eyes,* and a true children's book series *Frankie the Walk 'N Roll Dog.* She is a passionate advocate for dogs with Intervertebral Disc Disease (IVDD) and dogs in wheelchairs, as well as helping others see their challenges in a positive way.

WEB	www.joyfulpaws.com
FACEBOOK	www.facebook.com/joyfulpaws
	www.facebook.com/nationalwalknrolldogday
TWITTER	www.twitter.com/joyfulpaws

BECKI PACETTI has been in restaurant management for the last 25 years and hopes to retire from it in another ten. She is married to Michael Trotter, Jr and lives in Pearland, Texas; they have been together for nine years. She has two grown children, Amanda Merritt (34) and Jedidiah Merritt (30). Amanda has blessed Becki with a beautiful granddaughter, Emma Jeylene DeJesus, and they live in Peterborough, Ontario, Canada. Jedidiah lives in Destin, Florida. Becki has continued to care for her mother who has dementia for the last 3 years and will continue until the end of her Mom's life. Becki visits her mother about once a month to take care of any material things she needs, she cannot visit too long because her mom becomes very delusional after her visits. Becki knows that this is not her mom and still loves her very much and does all she can for her.

FACEBOOK	www.facebook.com/beckipacetti
TWITTER	www.twitter.com/pookiepacetti

ROBERT E. BONAFEDE has an A.S. in Marine Biology from Mitchell College in Connecticut and a B.A. in Economics from Bryant University in Rhode Island. He worked in the management field, and for more than 13 years as a full-time caregiver for his father. His hobbies are hiking, canoeing, skiing, swimming, working out and traveling. He also enjoys whale watching and dogs as pets. Bob hopes to do volunteer work helping others who may become caregivers, since he feels caregivers are not recognized for the work they do.

FACEBOOK	www.facebook.com/robert.bonafede.9

DR. ERICA KOSAL is a caregiver, public speaker, blogger and author of the book *Miracles for Daddy: A Family's Inspirational Fight against A Modern Medical Goliath*. She has been featured on ABC news, Care2.com, KidzEdge, Inspire Me Today and other media outlets. She is also a public speaker, inspiring people to take control of their own situation by adopting resilient strategies, and the blogger of *Traveling Troubled Times*, where she writes about her experiences and the strength of focusing on the good that can come from any situation. She and her husband (for whom she helps care as he battles for his health), maintain a website called *Bounce to Resilience*, designed to provide information and support to people experiencing extreme stress and adversity.

WEB	www.bouncetoresilience.com www.ericakosal.wordpress.com/
FACEBOOK	www.facebook.com/MiraclesforDaddy www.facebook.com/ekosal

LYNN GREENBLATT is a family caregiver for her husband, who has Complex Regional Pain Syndrome [CRPS], and a long-distance caregiver for her mother, who is rebuilding a new life after losing her beloved husband of 50 years almost 5 years ago. Caregiving began for Lynn when her father was diagnosed with multiple myeloma in December of 2007. As her father's condition deteriorated, her husband began to experience painful symptoms that took five months to diagnose. She became her husband's primary caregiver in 2008, shortly before her father passed away. Lynn's message to family caregivers is to reach out and use the resources available to them, to better manage caregiving, to create a Care Team to reduce stress and isolation, and to practice self-care in order to remain strong throughout their caregiving journey.

WEB	www.caregivingcafe.com/
	www.caregivingcafe.com/blog/
TWITTER	www.twitter.com/CaregivingCafe

MARK WILKINSON has been in the geophysical industry for 29 years. In that time he has held technical, management and senior management roles with a major oil company and geophysical service companies. Mark is a graduate of Texas A&M Department of Geophysics. He is married and has three children aged 22 (twins) and 16. From 1976-1982, Mark was caregiver of his father who had a stroke. From 1995-2003, he did the same when his mom also had a stroke. His role as caregiver for both his parents has taught him empathy for others facing life challenges. Now in his spare time, he's dabbled in a wide range of interests such as Civil War reenacting, hunting, fishing, cactus collecting, and recreational farming.

FACEBOOK	www.facebook.com/jmark.wilkinson1

MICHAEL RAY and his wife Deborah are simple people, born and raised in poverty in the south. He is a singer/songwriter praying to make a dime from it someday, and she is a brilliant, loyal wife who Michael says "tolerates a lot out of me and lives with little." He doesn't feel he would be the kind of man he is, nor would he have found his way back to God, without her in his life. She has stood by him for 20 years, and because he is completely disabled himself (as far as strenuous activity goes), he considers her his "caregiver." He has had heart and spinal problems that started a year after they were married and she has stood by him when many others would have sought greener pastures.

WEB	www.reverbnation.com/MichaelRay1ManShow
FACEBOOK	www.facebook.com/MichaelRayShow
	www.facebook.com/DeborahRobinson

SUZANNE ROSE spent many years in youth and family ministry. She went back to school later in life and holds a BA in Communication and an MA in Organizational Learning and Development. Her life turned a major corner when her husband experienced cardiac arrest and brain injury and was fully disabled, and she became his caregiver. She shares her story in the chapter "Riding into the Unknown" and as a contributing author to *Dancing through Life with Guts, Grace and Gusto: Fancy Footwork for the Woman's Sole.* After her husband's passing, she found that spiritual life coaching allowed her to integrate her experiences, education and work in a way to support and mentor others to make positive shifts and changes, move through blocks, old patterns and beliefs, to live the life they want to re-create with more passion, purpose and playfulness.

WEB	www.empoweringserenity.com
FACEBOOK	www.facebook.com/Empowering Serenity

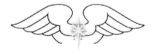

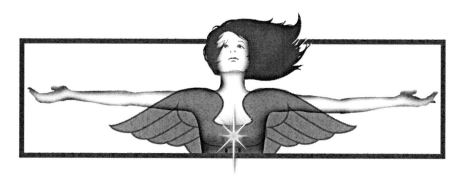

Special Patron of
Radiant Survivor

I would like to show my deepest appreciation and recognize the patron who made a very generous financial contribution to my book launch funding campaign, as well as promoted Radiant Survivor to the media: Pierpont Communications.

Pierpont Communications delivers cutting-edge, global public relations programming, marketing and digital expertise, and dynamic media counsel to bring our clients measurable results. They bring a level of senior leadership and fresh thinking to client engagements and emphasize becoming a partner, not just an advisor. They know their job is to objectively provide strategic counsel to clients, giving them the competitive edge to meet their goals.

To learn how Pierpont experience can drive the growth of your brand and business, visit them online at www.piercom.com.

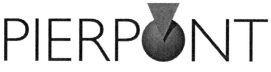

PUBLIC RELATIONS • PUBLIC AFFAIRS
INVESTOR RELATIONS • MARKETING

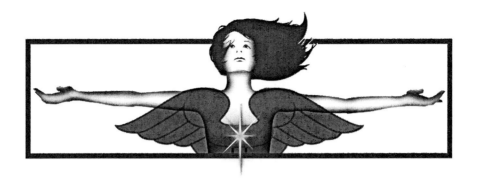

Books of Interest

These are some of the books I read in the time after my stroke that helped me on my road to healing and recovery. They showed me that life-altering experiences are truly treasures from heaven. This list also includes books written by some of the story contributors of *Radiant Survivor*, as well as the guest panelists of the Radiant Survivor telesummit that was held in November 2013.

Dallaire, Deny. *Many Shades of Green.* Dreamcatcher Publishing, 2010

Duane, Mal. *Alpha Chick.* Alpha Chick Press, 2011

Frederick, Sue. *Bridges to Heaven.* St. Martin's Press, 2013

Kosal, Dr. Erica. *Miracles for Daddy.* Burro Publishing, 2013

Kübler-Ross, Dr. Elisabeth. *On Death and Dying.* Scribner, 2013

Maslan, Allison. *Blast Off!* Morgan James Publishing, 2010

Moorjani, Anita. *Dying to Be Me.* Hay House, Inc., 2012

Mullins, Pamina. *Why Me?* Balboa Press International, 2011

Myss, Caroline. *Sacred Contracts.* Three Rivers Press, 2002

Occelli, Cynthia. *Resurrecting Venus.* Agape Media Int'l, LLC, 2012

Owen, Katherine T. Owen. *It's OK to Believe.* Presence Publishing, 2010

Perkins, John. *Shape Shifting.* Destiny Books, 1997

Perlmutter, Dr. David and Villoldo, Dr. Alberto. *Power up Your Brain.* Hay House, Inc., 2011

Ruiz, Don Miguel. *The Four Agreements.* Amber-Allen Publishing, 1997

Sablone, Aurelio. *From Geek to Chic.* Infinity Publishing, 2012

Scott, Deb. *The Sky is Green and The Grass is Blue.* AuthorHouse 2009

Siegel, Dr. Bernie. *The Art of Healing.* New World Library, 2013

Siegel, Dr. Bernie. *A Book of Miracles.* New World Library, 2011

Sorbo, Kevin. *True Strength.* Da Capo Press, 2011

Stephenson, Delanie. *The Calm before the Storm.* iUniverse, 2013

Taylor, Dr. Jill Bolte. *My Stroke of Insight.* Viking Penguin, a member of Penguin Group (USA) Inc., 2008

Techel, Barbara. *Through Frankie's Eyes.* Joyful Paw Prints, 2012

Tolle, Eckhart. *The Power of Now.* New World Library, 1999

Tucci, Erica. *Anything Is Possible.* Publish It Write, 2011

Weiss, Dr. Brian. *Many Lives, Many Masters.* Fireside, 1988

Weiss, Dr. Brian. *Miracles Happen.* HarperCollins, 2012

Whitelaw-Smith, Karen. *The Butterfly Experience.* Watkins Publishing, 2012

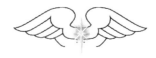

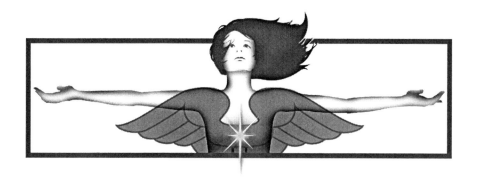

References

INTRODUCTION

1. Eckhart Tolle, *The Power of Now* (New World Library, 1999). P. 74

MY STORY

2. Dr. Brian Weiss, *Miracles Happen* (HarperCollins, 2012). p. 249
3. Erica Tucci, *Anything Is Possible* (Publish It Write, 2011), available at www.ericatucci.com/books
4. Eckhart Tolle, *The Power of Now* (New World Library, 1999). P. 86
5. Dr. Brian Weiss, *Miracles Happen* (HarperCollins, 2012). pp. 250, 251

YOU KNEW YOUR TRAUMA BEFORE YOU WERE BORN

6. Caroline Myss, *Sacred Contracts* (Three Rivers Press, 2002). p. 45
7. Ibid., pp. 111-112
8. Ibid., p. 113

9. See Aurelio's autobiographical memoir at
www.FromGeekToChicTheBook.com
10. Dr. Carl G. Jung, *Collected Works of C. G. Jung* (Princeton
University Press, 1958). vol. 7, p. 66

Limiting Beliefs:
What You Believe, You Receive

11. Ibid., vol. 11, pp. 447-448
12. Dr. Jill Bolte Taylor, *My Stroke of Insight* (Viking Penguin,
a member of Penguin Group (USA) Inc., 2008). p. 138
13. Ibid., pp. 32-33
14. Ibid., p. 140
15. Dr. David Perlmutter and Dr. Alberto Villoldo, *Power up
Your Brain* (Hay House, Inc., 2011). p. 78

Gratitude and Attitude

16. Quote by Melody Beattie at
http://www.melodybeattie.com

Establishing a Support System

17. Dr. Brian Weiss, *Miracles Happen* (HarperCollins, 2012).
pp. 13, 232

Surrendering – Letting Go and Letting God

18. Eckhart Tolle, *The Power of Now* (New World Library,
1999). pp. 205, 206
19. Quote by Cynthia Occelli – www.facebook.com/lifeblog
20. Quote by Madison Woods – www.madison-
woods.com/wordpress/philosophy-round-table-3/
21. Quote by Ellen Davis – www.huffingtonpost.com/ellen-
davis/surrender_b_1506604.html
22. Eckhart Tolle, *The Power of Now* (New World Library,
1999). P. 207

23. Ibid., p. 209

LIVING IN THE MOMENT

24. Ibid., p. 94
25. Ibid., p. 102

RECOVERY IS A PROCESS

26. Body Talk is a simple and effective holistic therapy that allows the body's energy systems to be re-synchronized so they can operate as nature intended.

MIRACLES DO HAPPEN

27. Dr. Brian Weiss, *Miracles Happen* (HarperCollins, 2012). p. 281

COMING FULL CIRCLE

28. Erica Tucci, *Anything Is Possible* (Publish It Write, 2011). p. 99
29. Richard Gordon, *Your Healing Hands* (North Atlantic Books, 1978). p. 123
30. "Pliér" means "to bend" in French; a plié is one of the first steps one learns in ballet.

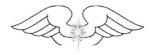

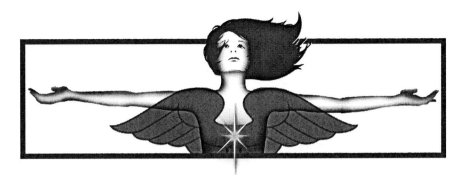

Other Books by Erica Tucci

Zesty Womanhood at 40 and Beyond: Second Act, New Role

Publish it Write, 2011
ISBN 978-0-9662451-3-4 (paperback);
ISBN 978-0-9662451-2-7 (e-book).

The sacred feminine is rising throughout the world like the Phoenix. *Zesty Womanhood at 40 and Beyond*, a spirited insightful book, invokes women to reclaim this Divine essence that is being reborn, first within themselves, and then to shine this beacon of the soul out into the Universe. It covers topics such as:

- Finding personal boundaries
- Experiencing love, the universal truth
- Seeing beauty through older eyes
- Transforming through relationships
- Reclaiming one's feminine power
- Letting go of old behaviors and thoughts
- Living a life without expectations
- From order to chaos...and back again
- Coming full circle

And what better way to bring it all to a close but through a few chuckles, as laughter is good for the soul.

The book also asks the reader to explore her own personal journey through exercises...to put the messages of each chapter into action.

Anything Is Possible

Publish it Write, 2011
ISBN 978-0-9662451-5-8 (paperback
ISBN 978-0-9662451-5-8 (e-book)

Based on a true story, this touching tale, traveling across time and space, reveals how love that appears unexpectedly and facing enormous obstacles can transform two people during the course of their relationship. Anything Is Possible will grip at the hearts of the readers, draw them into a deep inner conversation of compelling self-truths, and reveal how one woman, through these profound insights, was brought closer to her authentic essence within.

Through a professional interaction, Carla becomes entangled in an unexpected love affair. Emotionally torn by her seemingly impossible predicament of being in love with a married man with children living 5,000 miles away, how can she feel her way through the conflict between love and obligation, personal integrity and compromise? When love seems to triumph, a new battle ensues. Will the future be what she longs for? As she and her lover part ways in the end with an uncertainty of how all will work out, Carla is deeply saddened, yet feels a new sense of who she is and what she seeks in life as she ponders the rite of passage she has just moved through.

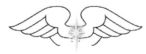

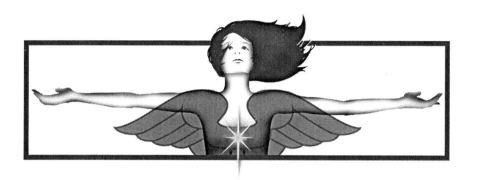

Connect with Erica Tucci

Web and Blogs

www.radiantsurvivor.com
www.ericatucci.com

Facebook

www.facebook.com/erica.tucci
www.facebook.com/RadiantSurvivor

Twitter:

@EricaTucciMuse

LinkedIn

www.linkedin.com/in/ericatucci

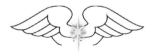

CPSIA information can be obtained at www.ICGtesting.com
Printed in the USA
LVOW08s1032291013

359076LV00002B/2/P

9 780966 245172